· Professi

MEDIZIN &
PHARMAZIE

Englisch-Deutsch
Deutsch-Englisch

Barbara Johnson

Compact Verlag

© 2002 Compact Verlag München
Alle Rechte vorbehalten. Nachdruck, auch auszugsweise,
nur mit ausdrücklicher Genehmigung des Verlages gestattet.
Chefredaktion: Ilse Hell
Redaktion: Alexandra Pawelczak, Julia Kotzschmar
Redaktionsassistenz: Ariane Busch, Nicole Weber
Fachredaktion: Kylie Robinson
Produktion: Martina Baur, Susana Spatz
Umschlaggestaltung: Inga Koch

ISBN: 3-8174-7517-9
7175171

Besuchen Sie uns im Internet: www.compactverlag.de

Vorwort

Das sichere Beherrschen des modernen Business English ist heute eine der wichtigsten Voraussetzungen für geschäftlichen und beruflichen Erfolg. Wer heute im Beruf weiterkommen will, muss mit internationalen Geschäftspartnern sicher kommunizieren sowie spezifisches Vokabular verstehen und anwenden können.

Dieses Nachschlagewerk bietet für den Fachbereich **Medizin und Pharmazie** eine kompetente und schnelle Hilfe in den verschiedensten Kommunikationssituationen. Das gezielt ausgewählte Fachvokabular wird durch zahlreiche, praxisnahe Beispiele in einen sprachlichen Zusammenhang gestellt.

Der **erste Teil** des Buches stellt die wesentlichen englischen Fachbegriffe in alphabetischer Reihenfolge dar. Jeder Eintrag wird übersetzt und mit Beispielsätzen und wichtigen Wortzusammensetzungen ergänzt. Im **zweiten Teil** finden Sie einen deutsch-englischen Wortschatzteil zum schnellen und sicheren Nachschlagen und Lernen. Zahlreiche nützliche Hinweise zu Sprachbesonderheiten, Landeskunde und der Geschäftswelt machen das Buch nicht nur im Büro, sondern auch auf Geschäftsreisen zu einem unverzichtbaren Nachschlagewerk.

Abkürzungen

adj	Adjektiv
adv	Adverb
jdm	jemandem
jdn	jemanden
jds	jemandes
jmd	jemand
n	Substantiv
pl	Plural
prep	Präposition
v	Verb
sb	somebody
sth	something

abdomen *n*
The abdomen is separated from the chest
and lungs by the diaphragm.
abdominal

Abdomen, Unterleib
Der Abdomen ist von der Brust und den
Lungen durch das Zwerchfell getrennt.
von dem Abdomen, Unterleibs-

ablutomania *n*
Patients suffering from ablutomania
never feel clean, however many showers
they take.

Waschzwang
Leute, die an einem Waschzwang leiden,
fühlen sich nie sauber, egal, wie oft sie
duschen.

abortion *n*
Abortion is still not allowed in some
countries.

Abtreibung
Abtreibung ist immer noch in manchen
Ländern verboten.

abscess *n*
An abscess may be caused by bacteria.

Abszess
Die Ursache eines Abszesses können
Bakterien sein.

absorption *n*
to absorb
Substances, such as forms of medication,
can be absorbed through the skin,
stomach and intestines.

Absorption
aufnehmen, absorbieren
Substanzen, wie z. B. Medikamente,
können durch die Haut, den Magen
und Darm aufgenommen werden.

abstinence n
Abstinence is the term used for patients
who deny themselves food, drink or
sexual intercourse.

Abstinenz
Abstinenz ist der Begriff für Patienten,
die auf Essen, Trinken oder Geschlechtsverkehr verzichten.

abuse *v*
The most common abused items are
drugs and alcohol.

missbrauchen
Am häufigsten Missbrauch wird mit
Drogen und Alkohol getrieben.

accident *n*
On the way home I witnessed a serious
car accident.

Unfall
Auf dem Heimweg war ich Zeuge eines
schweren Autounfalls.

accumulation *n*
The accumulation of acid in the blood
and body tissues causes the condition
referred to as acidosis.

Akkumulation
Die Akkumulation von Säure im Blut und
Gewebe verursacht Azidose.

accumulation of pus *n*
An accumulation of pus can occur when
a wound becomes infected.

Eiteransammlung
Eine Eiteransammlung kann vorkommen,
wenn eine Wunde infiziert wird.

acid *n*
Acid turns litmus paper red.

Säure
Lackmuspapier färbt sich bei Kontakt mit Säure rot.

acidity
acidosis

Säure, Säuregrad
Azidose

acne *n*
Teenagers often suffer from acne.

Akne
Jugendliche leiden oft an Akne.

acupuncture *n*
In recent years, acupuncture has become increasingly popular as an alternative to traditional Western medicine.

Akupunktur
Als Alternative zur traditionellen westlichen Medizin ist Akupunktur in den letzten Jahren immer beliebter geworden.

acute *n*
An acute illness is severe, and usually occurs suddenly.
acute delirium
acute ear

akut
Akute Krankheiten verlaufen heftig und treten für gewöhnlich plötzlich ein.
akutes Delirium
akute Mittelohrentzündung

Adam's apple *n*
When the thyroid cartilage is visible, it is referred to in layman's terms as the "Adam's apple".

Adamsapfel
Wenn der Schilddrüsenknorpel sichtbar ist, wird er in der Umgangssprache als „Adamsapfel" bezeichnet.

adaptation *n*
adapt
The eye adapts to the intensity of light.

Adaptation, Anpassung
anpassen, sich anpassen
Das Auge passt sich der Lichtintensität an.

additive *n*
Health food shops sell food free from additives and preservatives.

Zusatzstoff
Reformhäuser verkaufen Lebensmittel, die frei von Zusatzstoffen und Konservierungsmitteln sind.

adolescence *n*
Adolescence can be a difficult period in one's life.

Jugend
Die Jugend kann eine schwierige Zeit im Leben sein.

adrenalin *n*
Adrenalin is produced in stress situations.

Adrenalin
Adrenalin wird in Stresssituationen produziert.

aggression *n*
aggressive
Boys are sometimes more aggressive than girls.

Aggression
aggressiv
Jungs sind manchmal aggressiver als Mädchen.

albino *n*
An albino lacks pigmentation in the skin, eyes and hair.

Albino
Einem Albino fehlt die Pigmentierung von Haut, Augen und Haar.

alcohol *n*
alcoholism
Where is the borderline between heavy drinking and alcoholism?
Alcoholics Anonymous

Alkohol
Alkoholismus
Wo liegt die Grenze zwischen hohem Alkoholkonsum und Alkoholismus?
Anonyme Alkoholiker

aldehyde *n*
An aldehyde compound contains CHO.

Aldehyd
Eine Aldehydzusammensetzung enthält CHO.

alert *adj*
The patient was attentive and alert.

alert, rege, aufmerksam
Der Patient war aufmerksam und alert.

alleviate *v*
The painkillers will hopefully alleviate the symptoms.

lindern
Die Schmerzmittel werden hoffentlich die Symptome lindern.

amalgam *n*
In the last few years a lot of dental patients have had the amalgam fillings removed from their teeth.

Amalgam
In den letzten Jahren ließen sich viele Patienten das Amalgam aus ihren Zähnen entfernen.

ambulance *n*
The ambulance arrived at the scene of the accident.

Krankenwagen
Der Krankenwagen kam an der Unfallstelle an.

amenorrhoea *n*
There can be a number of reasons for amenorrhoea (when a woman does not menstruate).

Amenorrhoea
Amenorrhoea, d. h. das Ausbleiben der Regelblutung, kann eine Vielzahl an Ursachen haben.

amnesia *n*

People sometimes suffer from amnesia after a head injury.

Amnesie, Gedächtnisschwäche, Gedächtnisschwund
Nach einer Kopfverletzung leiden manche Leute an Gedächtnisschwund.

amoebic dysentery *n*
Amoebic dysentery is an inflammation of the intestines, more likely to be contracted in unhygienic conditions.

Amöbenruhr
Amöbenruhr ist eine Entzündung des Darmweges, die vorwiegend in unhygienischer Umgebung übertragen wird.

ampoule *n*
An ampoule is a small, sealed container which maintains liquids in a sterile condition.

Ampulle
Eine Ampulle ist ein kleines, versiegeltes Behältnis für die sterile Aufbewahrung von Flüssigkeiten.

anaemia *n*
I have suffered from anaemia all my life.

Anämie, Blutarmut
Ich habe mein Leben lang an Blutarmut gelitten.

---

analgesic *n*
An analgesic is a pain killer, which acts without the patient losing consciousness.

Analgetikum
Ein Analgetikum dient als Schmerzmittel, ohne dass der Patient bewusstlos wird.

---

anamnesis *n*
The medical history of a patient is the anamnesis.

Anamnese
Die medizinische Geschichte eines Patienten bezeichnet man als Anamnese.

---

aneurysm *n*
An aneurysm is the sac formed when the wall of a blood vessel dilates.

Aneurysma
Ein Aneurysma ist eine sackförmige Ausweitung einer Arterie.

---

angina *n*
An attack of angina can involve choking.

angina of effort
anginoid

Angina
Bei einer Angina können Erstickungssymptome auftreten.
Effort-Syndrom
anginaartig

---

angina pectoris *n*

Angina Pectoris

---

anorexia *n*
Teenage girls are often susceptible to anorexia.

Anorexie
Mädchen im Teenageralter sind anfällig für Anorexie.

---

antacid *n*
An antacid neutralises the overproduction of acid in the stomach.

Antazidum
Ein Antazidum neutralisiert die Überproduktion von Säure im Magen.

---

antibiotic *n*
When I was a child I was often prescribed antibiotics against insect bites.

Antibiotikum
Als ich ein Kind war, wurden mir oft Antibiotika gegen Insektenstiche verschrieben.

---

anti-coagulant *n*

An anti-coagulant prevents the blood from clotting.

Antikoagulans, gerinnungshemmende Substanz
Ein Antikoagulans wirkt gerinnungshemmend.

---

antidepressant *n*
An antidepressant is prescribed to patients suffering from depression, sometimes to reduce fear, or as a stimulant.

Antidepressivum
Ein Antidepressivum wird Patienten mit Depressionen verschrieben, um ihre Angst zu verringern oder sie aufzuheitern.

antidote *n*
He was bitten by a snake and lucky that the antidote was available.

Antidot, Gegengift
Er wurde von einer Schlange gebissen; glücklicherweise war das Gegengift gleich zur Hand.

antihistamine *n*
Antihistamine tablets alleviate the symptoms of allergies.

Antihistaminikum
Antihistaminika schwächen die Symptome von Allergien ab.

anti-inflammatory *adj*

The tablets have an anti-inflammatory effect and should be taken regularly.

entzündungshemmend, antiinflammatorisch
Die Tabletten wirken entzündungshemmend und sollen regelmäßig eingenommen werden.

antiseptic *adj*
The child had grazed his knee, so his mother put some antiseptic ointment on it.

antiseptisch
Das Kind hatte sich das Knie aufgeschürft; die Mutter behandelte es daraufhin mit einer antiseptischen Salbe.

antiseptic *n*
She bought an antiseptic cream at the chemist's.

antiseptisch, keimtötend
Sie kaufte eine antiseptische Salbe in der Apotheke.

aphasia *n*
Aphasia is caused by injury to the brain centres.

Aphasie
Aphasie entsteht durch Verletzung der Gehirnzentren.

apoplexy *n*

Paralysis often succeeds apoplexy.

Apoplexie, Gehirnschlag, Hirnschlag
Nach einem Gehirnschlag folgen oft Lähmungen.

appendix *n*
appendicitis
My neighbour was rushed into hospital with appendicitis.
to ligate the appendix

Appendix, Blinddarm
Appendizitis
Mein Nachbar wurde mit Appendizitis als Notfall ins Krankenhaus eingeliefert.
den Wurmfortsatz abbinden

applicator *n*
An applicator is a device which makes it easier to use or take medication.

Applikator
Ein Applikator macht es einfacher, Medikamente anzuwenden oder einzunehmen.

approve *v*
approved
In the United States new drugs have to be approved by the FDA (Food and Drugs Administration).

zulassen
zugelassen
In den Vereinigten Staaten müssen neue Medikamente von der FDA (Administration für Lebensmittel und Drogen) zugelassen werden.

areola *n*

The areola is either the circular area around the nipple or the inflamed area around a pimple.

Warzenvorhof, Inflammation rund um einen Pickel
Das englisch Wort „aerola" bezieht sich entweder auf den Warzenvorhof oder auf den entzündeten Hautfleck um einen Pickel.

armpit *n*

People used to take temperatures by placing the thermometer under the patient's armpit.

Achsel
Früher hat man Fieber unter dem Arm des Patienten gemessen.

arrest *v*

The doctors prescribed drugs which were intended to arrest the growth of the tumour.
cardiac arrest

hemmen, stoppen
Die Ärzte verschrieben Medikamente, die den Wachstum des Tumors hemmen sollten.
Herzstillstand

arsenic *n*

The use of arsenic as a means of murder by poisoning, is popular in detective novels.
arsenic paralysis

Arsen
In Detektivromanen ist Arsen ein beliebtes Mordinstrument.

Arsenlähmung

arteriosclerosis *n*

My aunt has been suffering from arteriosclerosis for the past few years now.

Arteriosklerose
Meine Tante leidet nun schon seit einigen Jahren an Arteriosklerose.

artery *n*

The arteries lead away from the heart.
arterial

Arterie, Schlagader
Die Arterien führen vom Herzen weg.
arteriell

arthritis *n*

One of my pupils suffers from arthritis and has difficulty writing.

Arthritis, Gelenkentzündung
Einer meiner Schüler leidet an Arthritis und hat dadurch Schwierigkeiten beim Schreiben.

arthroscopy *n*

An arthroscopy was performed to examine Mrs Paul's joints.

Arthroskopie
Eine Arthroskopie wurde durchgeführt, um die Gelenke von Frau Paul zu untersuchen.

artificial *adj*
artificial insemination
The baby was conceived by artificial insemination.
artificial respiration
artificial teeth
artificial ventilation

künstlich
künstliche Befruchtung
Das Baby wurde durch künstliche Befruchtung empfangen.
künstliche Beatmung
künstliche Zähne
künstliche Beatmung

aseptic *n*
You need to ensure an aseptic environment.

keimfrei
Du musst eine keimfreie Umgebung sichern.

asthma *n*

Asthma

Asthma patients suffer from sudden attacks of breathlessness (and coughing) caused by narrowing of the bronchial tubes. The causes can be allergies, infection or exertion.

astringent *adj*
An astringent lotion has an invigorating effect on the skin, causing skin tissue to contract.

adstringierend
Eine adstringierende Lotion wirkt belebend auf die Haut; sie bewirkt das Zusammenziehen des Hautgewebes.

athlete's foot *n*
Athlete's foot is a condition often found between the toes.

Fußpilz
Fußpilz findet sich oft zwischen den Zehen.

atrial *adj*
atrium

Vorhof...
Vorhof

atrophy *n*
We speak of atrophy when an organ fails to grow to the normal size, or wastes away.

Rückbildung
Wir reden von einer Rückbildung, wenn ein Organ seine normale Größe nicht erreicht oder an Masse verliert.

attack *n*
heart attack
The death rate as a result of heart attack is very high in western society.

to control an attack

Anfall
Herzinfarkt
Die Todesrate als Folge eines Herzinfarktes ist in der westlichen Bevölkerung sehr hoch.
einen Anfall behandeln

attending physician *n*
I consulted the attending physician.

behandelnder Arzt
Ich erkundigte mich beim behandelnden Arzt.

audio-frequency *n*
Sound waves of an audio-frequency of 20–20,000 hertz are audible to the human ear.

Taktfrequenz
Schallwellen mit einer Taktfrequenz von 20 bis 20.000 Hertz sind vom menschlichen Ohr wahrnehmbar.

auscultate *n*
To auscultate is to listen to the patient's body with a stethoscope.

Abhorchen
Der Vorgang des Abhorchens bedeutet, die Geräusche des Körpers mit einem Stethoskop abzuhören.

autism *n*
autistic
Autistic children do not react to their environment.

Autismus
autistisch
Autistische Kinder reagieren nicht auf ihre Umwelt.

autopsy *n*
An autopsy was performed to determine the cause of death.

Autopsie
Eine Autopsie wurde durchgeführt, um die Todesursache festzustellen.

available *adj*
available on prescription only
The doctor recommended some specific tablets which are available on prescription only.

verfügbar
verschreibungspflichtig
Der Arzt empfahl besondere Tabletten, die verschreibungspflichtig sind.

axillary hair *n*
Women often remove axillary hair.

Achselhaar
Frauen entfernen oft ihr Achselhaar.

B

babble *v*
Babies babble before they learn to talk.

lallen
Babys lallen, bevor sie sprechen lernen.

babyfood *n*
Babyfood is available in various different forms.

Säuglingsnahrung
Säuglingsnahrung ist in verschiedenen Formen erhältlich.

babysitter *n*

Babysitter, Kinderbetreuung

Bach flowers *n*

Bachblüten

Dr. Edward Bach, a British doctor, developed the use of **Bach flowers** in treating patients in the 1930's in Oxfordshire, England. "Our work is steadfastly to adhere to the simplicity and purity of this method of healing," were his words in 1936.

bacillus *n*
A bacillus is a rod-shaped bacterium.

Bazillus
Ein Bazillus ist ein stäbchenförmiges Bakterium.

back *n*
backache
Pregnant women are prone to suffer from backache.
flat on one's back
back of the hand

Rücken
Rückenschmerzen
Schwangere Frauen leiden meist an Rückenschmerzen.
bettlägerig
Handrücken

bacteria *n*
Bacteria are only visible under a microscope.

Bakterien
Bakterien sind nur unter einem Mikroskop sichtbar.

bad breath *n*
Bad breath can have various causes.

Mundgeruch
Mundgeruch kann verschiedene Ursachen haben.

bag *n*
A bag is used to collect urine or other bodywaste, when a patient's organs are no longer able to do so, either temporarily or permanently.

bag change procedure

Beutel
Ein Beutel wird eingesetzt, um Urin oder andere Exkremente zu sammeln, wenn die hierfür zuständigen Organe des Patienten dazu entweder vorübergehend oder dauerhaft nicht mehr in der Lage sind.
Beutelwechsel

balance *n*
Balance is both the body equilibrium and the stability of the emotions.
well-balanced

Gleichgewicht
Gleichgewicht meint sowohl körperliche als auch emotionale Stabilität.
ausgeglichen

bald *adj*
Some men become bald at an early age.
baldness

kahl
Einige Männer werden früh kahl.

Kahlheit

ball-and-socket joint *n*
The upper arm is connected to the shoulder by a ball-and-socket joint.
ball-and-socket prosthesis

Kugelgelenk
Der Oberarm ist durch ein Kugelgelenk mit der Schulter verbunden.
Kugelprothese

balm *n*
Balm is an aromatic, soothing ointment used in healing.

Balsam
Balsam ist eine evtl. aromatische, beruhigende Salbe, die als Heilmittel eingesetzt wird.

bandage *n*
Car first-aid kits contain a variety of bandages in different sizes.

Verband
Erste-Hilfe-Kästen in PKWs enthalten eine Auswahl von Verbandsrollen verschiedener Größen.

barber's rash *n*
Barber's rash occurs on the bearded part of the neck and face in men.

Bartflechte
Bartflechte tritt bei Männern in der Bartgegend auf.

barbiturate *n*
Barbiturates are used as sedatives.

Barbiturat
Barbiturate werden als Schlafmittel eingesetzt.

Bartholin's gland *n*
Bartholin's glands are two small glands which produce a lubricant during sexual stimulation.

Bartholin-Drüse
Die Bartholin-Drüsen sind zwei kleine Drüsen, die bei sexueller Erregung ein Gleitsekret erzeugen.

basic need *n*
The basic needs of humans are food, clothes and shelter.

Grundbedürfnis
Die Grundbedürfnisse eines Menschen sind Nahrung, Kleidung und Herberge.

basic substance *n*
basic value

Grundsubstanz
Grundwert

basilar *adj*
basilar artery
basilar membrane
basilar meningitis

Basis
Basilaris
Basilarmembran
Basilarmeningitis

bath salts *n*
Taking a long bath containing fragrant bath salts is very relaxing.

Badezusätze
Ein langes Bad mit duftenden Badezusätzen ist sehr entspannend.

beauty spot *n*
A mole or similar mark on a woman's face is sometimes called a beauty spot.

Schönheitsfleck
Ein Leberfleck oder ein ähnlicher Fleck im Gesicht einer Frau wird manchmal als Schönheitsfleck bezeichnet.

bedsore *n*
Bedsores are caused by having to lie in bed for an abnormal length of time due to illness.

wundgelegene Stelle
Patienten liegen sich wund, wenn sie aufgrund einer Krankheit für eine sehr lange Zeit ans Bett gefesselt sind.

behaviour *n*
behaviour pattern
Research scientists study the behaviour patterns of animals.

Verhalten
Verhaltensmuster
Wissenschaftler beobachten die Verhaltensmuster von Tieren.

belladonna *n*
Belladonna is obtained from deadly nightshade.

Tollkirsche
Belladonna wird von der Tollkirsche gewonnen.

belly button *n*
"Belly button" is the popular word for "navel".

Bauchnabel
Im Englischen ist „belly button" der umgangssprachliche Ausdruck für Bauchnabel.

benign *adj*
This tumour is benign.
benignancy

gutartig
Dieser Tumor ist gutartig.
Gutartigkeit

bereavement *n*
Bereavement is when someone has lost a loved one.

Trauerfall
Es wird als Trauerfall bezeichnet, wenn jemand eine geliebte Person verloren hat.

beta-blocker *n*
Beta-blockers reduce the secretion of adrenalin, and are used to treat high-blood pressure or heart disease.

Betablocker
Betablocker vermindern die Produktion von Adrenalin und werden gegen hohen Blutdruck oder Herzkrankheiten eingesetzt.

betacarotene *n*
The body converts betacarotene into vitamin A.

Betacarotin
Der Körper wandelt Betacarotin in Vitamin A um.

bifocal glasses n pl
Bifocal glasses enable the wearer to read without changing glasses.

Zweistärkenbrille
Die Zweistärkenbrille erspart beim Lesen das Wechseln der Brille.

bile *n*
The liver produces bile, which is then stored in the gall bladder.
biliary duct
bile-stone
bile-trouble

Galle, Gallenflüssigkeit
Die Leber produziert Gallenflüssigkeit, die dann in der Galle gespeichert wird.
Gallengang
Gallenstein
Gallenleiden

biopsy *n*
A biopsy, the examination of tissue under a microscope, is carried out in order to ascertain the extent of a disease.

Biopsie
Eine Biopsie, d. h. die Untersuchung von Gewebe unter einem Mikroskop, wird durchgeführt, um die Beschaffenheit einer Krankheit festzustellen.

biopsy *n*
The removal of microscopic quantities of tissue for diagnostic purposes is referred to as a biopsy.

Biopsie
Die Entfernung mikroskopischer Mengen von Gewebe zu diagnostischen Zwecken wird Biopsie bezeichnet.

biotype *n*
A biotype is a sub-group of any species.

Biotyp
Ein Biotyp ist eine Untergruppe einer Spezie.

biped *n*
The word "biped" is derived from the Latin meaning "two feet", and refers to two-legged animals.

Zweibeiner
Das englische Wort „biped" kommt aus dem Lateinischen und bezeichnet Tiere mit zwei Beinen.

birth certificate *n*
A birth certificate is issued by the appropriate authority following the birth of a baby.

Geburtsurkunde
Eine Geburtsurkunde wird nach der Geburt eines Babys vom zuständigen Amt ausgestellt.

birth control *n*
birth control pill
There are a number of alternatives to the birth control pill.

Geburtenkontrolle
Antibabypille
Es gibt einige Alternativen zur Antibabypille.

birth mark *n*
A birthmark is so-named because it is already present at birth.

Muttermal
Ein Muttermal wird im Englischen als „birthmark" bezeichnet, weil es schon bei der Geburt vorhanden ist.

bismuth *n*
Bismuth compounds are used in medicine.

Wismut
Zusammensetzungen aus Wismut werden in der Medizin eingesetzt.

blackhead *n*
Blackheads are clogged pores or ducts.

Mitesser
Mitesser sind verstopfte Poren oder Kanäle.

blade *n*
A scalpel has a short, thin blade.

Klinge
Ein Skalpell hat eine kurze, dünne Klinge.

bland diet *n*
Patients with stomach problems are prescribed a bland diet.

Schonkost
Patienten mit Magenproblemen wird Schonkost verschrieben.

bleed to death *v*
The accident happened on a deserted road and the car driver bled to death.

verbluten
Der Unfall passierte auf einer selten befahrenen Straße und so verblutete der Autofahrer.

bleeding *n*
The people at the scene of the car accident attended to the injured, and attempted to stop the bleeding.
bleeding time

Blutung
Die Personen an der Unfallstelle kümmerten sich um die Verletzten und versuchten, ihre Blutungen zu stillen.
Blutungszeit

blemish *n*
She wishes to have a blemish removed from her face.

Schönheitsfehler
Sie möchte einen Schönheitsfehler in ihrem Gesicht entfernt haben.

blind liver biopsy *n*
A blind liver biopsy is performed in order to be able to examine tissue from this area.

Leberblindpunktion
Eine Leberblindpunktion wird durchgeführt, um Gewebe aus diesem Bereich zu untersuchen.

blister *n*
Wearing new or ill-fitting shoes can cause blisters.

Hautblase
Das Tragen von neuen oder schlecht passenden Schuhen kann Blasen verursachen.

bloated feeling *n*

Flatulence causes a bloated feeling in the lower abdomen.

mit Darmblähungen assoziiertes Gefühl von Unwohlsein
Darmblähungen verursachen ein aufgeblähtes Gefühl im Unterleib.

blood corpuscle *n*
Red blood corpuscles contain haemoglobin and transport oxygen and carbon dioxide; white blood corpuscles protect the body against disease.
blood donor

Blutkörperchen
Rote Blutkörperchen enthalten Hämoglobin und transportieren Sauerstoff sowie Kohlendioxid; weiße Blutkörperchen schützen den Körper vor Krankheiten.
Blutspender

blood drawing set *n*
A blood drawing set is used to extract blood.

Blutentnahmeset
Ein Blutentnahmeset wird bei der Blutabnahme verwendet.

blood group *n*

Blutgruppe

blood *n*
Blood has many functions, one of which is to supply the body with oxygen from the lungs.
blood bank
blood count

Blut
Blut hat viele Funktionen. Eine davon besteht darin, Sauerstoff von den Lungen zum restlichen Körper zu transportieren.
Blutbank
Blutbild

blood pack *n*
A blood pack contains blood to be used in a transfusion.

Blutbeutel
Ein Blutbeutel enthält Blut für eine Transfusion.

blood poisoning *n*
Blood poisoning occurs when a local infection spreads through the body via the lymphatic system and blood vessels.

Blutvergiftung
Blutvergiftungen entstehen durch die Verbreitung einer lokalen Infektion im Körper über das lymphatische System und die Blutgefäße.

blood pressure *n*

Blutdruck

blood sugar *n*
blood sugar level
The blood sugar level is the amount of glucose present in the blood.

Blutzucker
Blutzuckerspiegel
Der Blutzuckerspiegel bezeichnet die Menge an Glukose, die im Blut vorhanden ist.

blood test *n*

Blutprobe

blood transfusion *n*
A blood transfusion is carried out when a patient has lost too much blood.

Bluttransfusion
Eine Bluttransfusion wird durchgeführt, wenn ein Patient zu viel Blut verloren hat.

blood vessels *n*

Blutgefäße

body *n*
Medicine is concerned with the health of body and mind.
body fluid
body orifice
body posture
body sense
body weight

Körper
Die Medizin befasst sich mit der Gesundheit des Körpers und des Geistes.
Körperflüssigkeit
Körperöffnung
Körperhaltung
Körperempfinden
Körpergewicht

bolus injection *n*
An injection containing a large quantity of a drug is a bolus injection.

Bolusinjektion
Die Injektion einer hochdosierten Droge ist eine Bolusinjektion.

bone marrow *n*
bone marrow transplantation
Donors are sought for bone marrow transplants.
bone softening
bone tissue

Knochenmark
Knochenmarktransplantation
Es werden Spender für Knochenmarktransplantationen gesucht.
Knochenerweichung
Knochengewebe

bone *n*
bone cancer
bone cartilage
bone deformity
bone fracture
Older women suffering from bone loss are more prone to bone fractures, should they fall.
bone growth
bone deposit
bone loss

Knochen
Knochenkrebs
Knochenknorpel
Knochendeformität
Knochenbruch
Ältere Frauen, die an Knochenschwund leiden, sind bei Stürzen anfällig für Knochenbrüche.
Knochenwachstum
Knochenablagerung
Knochenschwund

borderline *n*
When it is difficult to decide exactly how serious an illness is, we speak of a "borderline" case.

Grenzlinie
Wenn es schwierig ist, über die Einordnung einer Krankheit zu entscheiden, reden wir von einem „Grenzfall".

bottle-feeding *n*
Babies often object when mothers want to change from breast to bottle-feeding!

Ernährung mit der Flasche
Babys wehren sich meist, wenn die Mutter vom Stillen auf Flaschenernährung wechselt.

bowel evacuation *n*
Nurses always ask patients if bowel evacuation has taken place.

Stuhlgang
Krankenschwestern fragen immer nach dem Stuhlgang.

bowel obstruction *n*

Darmverschluss

brace *n* *Children often have to wear a brace.*	**Zahnspange** *Kinder müssen oft eine Zahnspange tragen.*
brachial vein *n* *The brachial vein is the arm vein.*	**Armvene** *Das englische Wort „brachial" beschreibt hier die Armvene.*
braille *n*	**Blindenschrift**

The French inventor, musician and teacher of the blind, **Louis Braille**, 1809 – 1852, invented a system of raised writing for the blind, which was named after him. He himself had become blind when he was three years old.

brain death *n*	**Hirntod**

Brain death is usually described as the actual point of death, when brain damage causes the patient to stop breathing. The heart may be attached to a mechanical ventilator and continue to beat.

brain *n* **brain axis** **brain concussion** *The man was taken to hospital after the accident, because he was suffering from (brain) concussion.*	**Gehirn** **Hirnstamm** **Gehirnerschütterung** *Der Mann wurde nach dem Unfall ins Krankenhaus eingeliefert, weil er an einer Gehirnerschütterung litt.*
brain tumour *n* *The specialist diagnosed a brain tumour.*	**Gehirntumor** *Der Spezialist stellte einen Gehirntumor fest.*
break down *v* *After the death of her husband she suffered a nervous breakdown.*	**zusammenbrechen** *Nach dem Tod ihres Mannes erlitt sie einen Nervenzusammenbruch.*
breast *n* **breastfeed** *I breastfed my son for nearly a year.* **breast cancer** **breast palpitation**	**Brustdrüse** **stillen** *Ich stillte meinen Sohn fast ein Jahr lang.* **Brustkrebs** **Abtasten der Brust**
breath *n* **breathlessness** *One of the symptoms the patient complained of was breathlessness.*	**Atem, Atemzug** **Atemnot** *Der Patient klagt u. a. über Atemnot.*

breech delivery *n*
After examining the mother, the doctors were expecting a breech delivery.

Geburt bei Steißlage
Die Ärzte untersuchten die Mutter und stellten die Steißlage des Kindes fest.

bridge *n*
The dentist extracted the tooth and recommended a bridge as the best solution.

Zahnbrücke
Der Zahnarzt zog den Zahn und empfahl eine Brücke als beste Lösung.

broad-shouldered *adj*
The patient was a broad-shouldered man.

breitschultrig
Der Patient war ein breitschultriger Mann.

broad-spectrum antibiotic *n*
A broad-spectrum antibiotic has different uses.

Breitband-Antibiotikum
Ein Breitband-Antibiotikum hat ein weitreichendes Anwendungsfeld.

bromine *n*
Bromine is a pungent red liquid which is used in the production of chemicals.

Brom
Brom ist eine stark riechende, rote Flüssigkeit, die bei der Produktion von Chemikalien verwendet wird.

bronchia n pl
The term "bronchia" refers to the bronchi and the smaller branches extending from them.

Bronchien
Als Bronchien werden sowohl die Hauptzweige der Trachea als auch die kleineren Abzweigungen bezeichnet.

bronchioles *n*
The bronchioles are the smaller bronchial tubes which terminate in alveoli.

Bronchiolen
Die Bronchiolen sind kleinere Röhrchen, die in den Alveolen enden.

Bronchitis *n*
Bronchitis is a disease of the lungs caused by inflammation of the bronchial mucous membranes.

Bronchitis
Bronchitis ist eine Lungenerkrankung, die auf die Entzündung der Bronchienschleimhaut zurückzuführen ist.

bronchoscope *n*
A bronchoscope is used for examining the bronchial tubes.
bronchoscopy

Bronchoskop
Ein Bronchoskop wird zur Untersuchung der Bronchien verwendet.
Bronchoskopie

bruise *n*
The man was lucky to have escaped with only minor cuts and bruises.

Bluterguss
Der Mann hatte Glück, mit nur leichten Schnittwunden und Blutergüssen davongekommen zu sein.

budget *n*
The hospital budget was limited.

Haushaltsplan, Haushaltsmittel
Die Haushaltsmittel des Krankenhauses waren beschränkt.

buffer solution *n*
A buffer solution contains an ionic compound and has a stable pH.

Pufferlösung
Eine Pufferlösung enthält eine ionische Zusammensetzung und hat einen stabilen pH-Wert.

bulbous nose *n*
The man consulted the specialist about his bulbous nose, because it made him feel unsure of himself.

Knollennase
Der Mann konsultierte wegen seiner Knollennase einen Spezialisten, weil er sich unsicher fühlte.

bulimia *n*
Bulimia sufferers compulsively overeat and then vomit.

Bulimie, Ess-Brechsucht
An Bulimie leidende Menschen essen zwangsmäßig zuviel und erbrechen danach.

burn *n*
After the accident several people were taken to hospital suffering from burns.

burn shock

Verbrennung, Brandwunde
Nach dem Unfall wurden einige Leute mit Brandwunden ins Krankenhaus gebracht.
Verbrennungsschock

butterfly fracture *n*
The child had a butterfly fracture.

butterfly shaped vertebrae

Schmetterlingsbruch
Das Kind hatte einen Schmetterlingsbruch.
Schmetterlingswirbel

buttocks *n*
Buttocks are the muscular tissue forming the human rump.

Gesäß
Das Gesäß besteht aus muskulösem Gewebe.

buzzing *n*
She complained to the ENT specialist of a buzzing in her left ear.

Ohrensausen
Sie klagte beim Hals-Nasen-Ohren-Arzt über Ohrensausen im linken Ohr.

bypass *n*
Bypass surgery redirects the blood flow to avoid diseased tissue.

Bypass
Eine Bypass-Operation leitet das Blut um und umgeht somit krankes Gewebe.

C

candidiasis *n*
Candidiasis is an infection with the Candida fungus.

Candidiasis
Candidiasis ist eine Infizierung durch den Candida-Fungus.

carcinoma *n*
The carcinoma gave rise to metastases.

Karzinom, bösartige Geschwulst
Durch das Karzinom bildeten sich Metastasen.

caries *n*
 Caries can lead to abscesses and the loss of the tooth.
 caries of dental enamel

Karies
 Karies kann zu einem Abszess und zum Verlust des Zahnes führen.
 Zahnschmelzkaries

cerebellum *n*
 The functions of the cerebellum are the coordination of voluntary movements and maintenance of balance.

Cerebellum, Kleinhirn
 Die Funktionen des Cerebellum sind die Koordination von volontären Bewegungen sowie das Erhalten des Gleichgewichts.

cerumen *n*
 She had an excessive amount of cerumen, or earwax, in her left ear.

Cerumen, Ohrenschmalz
 Sie hatte eine übermäßige Menge an Ohrenschmalz im linken Ohr.

chemotherapy *n*
 Chemotherapy is often used against cancer.

Chemotherapie
 Chemotherapie wird gegen Krebs eingesetzt.

chloasma n (chloasmata pl)
 A chloasma is a yellowish-brown mark on the face, which can have various causes including pregnancy, the contraceptive pill or liver disease.

Chloasma
 Ein Chloasma ist ein gelbbrauner Fleck im Gesicht, der verschiedene Ursachen haben kann, wie z. B. Schwangerschaft, Antibabypille oder Leberkrankheiten.

cholera *n*
 The Asiatic variety of cholera can prove deadly.

Cholera
 Die asiatische Variante von Cholera kann tödlich sein.

cholesterol *n*
 A high level of cholesterol in the blood may lead to artheriosclerosis and subsequently to heart disease.

Cholesterin
 Ein hoher Cholesterinspiegel kann zur Arteriosklerose und anschließend zu Herzkrankheiten führen.

chromosome *n*
 A chromosome is one of the rod-shaped structures in the cell nucleus which contains hereditary factors.

Chromosom
 Ein Chromosom ist eine stäbchenförmige Struktur im Zellkern, die Erbfaktoren enthält.

chronic bronchitis *n*

chronische Bronchitis

If an attack of bronchitis is not completely healed, the illness can recur in a chronic form, **chronic bronchitis,** especially in unfavourable weather conditions, such as a damp, cold British winter.

coated pill *n*
 Coated pills are easier to swallow.

Dragee
 Dragees sind einfach zu schlucken.

coccyx *n*
The coccyx is a vestigial tail at the base of the spinal column.

Steißbein
Das Steißbein ist ein kleiner Knochen am Ende der Wirbelsäule.

codeine *n*
Codeine is a drug prepared from morphine and used as a sedative.

Kodein
Kodein ist eine aus Morphium erzeugte Droge, die als Schlafmittel eingesetzt wird.

cod-liver oil *n*
Cod-liver oil is rich in vitamins A and D.

Lebertran
Lebertran ist reich an Vitamin A und D.

cold *n*
I usually catch colds in the autumn, when the weather is changeable.
cold shock
cold sore

Erkältung
Ich erkälte mich normalerweise im Herbst, wenn das Wetter wechselhaft ist.
Kälteschock
Gesichtsherpes

colic *n*
Some babies have colic during the first three months after birth.

Kolik
Manche Babys bekommen während der ersten drei Monate nach der Geburt eine Kolik.

coliform bacteria n pl
Coliform bacteria are present in the intestines.

Kolibakterien
Kolibakterien sind im Darm vorhanden.

colon *n*
The colon is part of the large intestine.

Dickdarm
Der Dickdarm ist ein Teil des Darmweges.

colostomy *n*
When performing a colostomy a surgeon creates an opening from the colon to the surface of the body.

Kolostomie
Wenn ein Chirurg eine Kolostomie durchführt, macht er eine Öffnung vom Dickdarm zur Körperoberfläche.

colostrum *n*
The first fluid a baby receives from the breast after birth is the colostrum.

Vormilch
Die erste Flüssigkeit, die ein Baby nach der Geburt von der Brust bekommt, ist die Vormilch.

colour blind *adj*
People who are colour-blind have difficulty distinguishing between certain colours, such as red and green.

farbenblind
Farbenblinde Personen haben Schwierigkeiten, zwischen bestimmten Farben zu unterscheiden, wie zum Beispiel zwischen rot und grün.

coma *n*
The man lay in a coma for a number of weeks.

Koma
Der Mann lag mehrere Wochen im Koma.

comatose *adj*
She was comatose after the accident.

komatös, bewusstlos
Sie war nach dem Unfall bewusstlos.

commit suicide *v*
My friend attempted to commit suicide by taking an overdose of sleeping pills.

Selbstmord begehen
Meine Freundin versuchte Selbstmord zu begehen, indem sie eine Überdosis Schlaftabletten einnahm.

company physician *n*
Larger companies often have a company physician.

Betriebsarzt
Größere Firmen haben oft einen Betriebsarzt.

comparative psychology *n*
Comparative psychology looks at the behaviour of different species, comparing similarities and differences.

Komparative Psychologie
Die Komparative Psychologie betrachtet das Verhalten verschiedener Arten und sucht Ähnlichkeiten sowie Unterschiede.

complexion *n*
The patient had a very pale complexion.

Teint
Die Patientin war sehr blass.

complicated fracture *n*
A friend of mine was in a motorcycle accident and the doctors diagnosed a complicated fracture of the tibia.

Trümmerbruch
Ein Freund von mir war in einen Motorradunfall verwickelt und die Ärzte stellten einen Trümmerbruch des Schienbeins fest.

complications *n*
The old lady only had a cold, but then there were complications and she had to go into hospital.

Komplikationen
Die ältere Frau war zunächst nur erkältet; doch dann sind Komplikationen aufgetreten und sie musste ins Krankenhaus.

compress *n*
She firmly applied a cold compress to the painful area.

Kompresse
Sie drückte eine kalte Kompresse fest auf die schmerzhafte Stelle.

compulsion *n*
The German psychiatric patient who has a compulsion performs trivial repetitive actions against his own will.

Zwang
Der deutsche Patient in der Psychiatrie, der unter einem Zwang leidet, wiederholt unwichtige Aufgaben gegen seinen eigenen Willen.

compulsory hospitalisation *n*
Compulsory hospitalisation is most likely to apply to psychiatric patients.

Zwangseinweisung
Die Zwangseinweisung trifft überwiegend bei Patienten in der Psychiatrie zu.

computerized tomography *n*
Computerized tomography enables the three-dimensional examination of areas of the body.

Computertomographie
Computertomographie ermöglicht die dreidimensionale Untersuchung von Körperregionen.

confused *adj*
The driver was able to get out of the car after the accident, but he was confused.

verwirrt
Der Autofahrer konnte nach dem Unfall zwar aussteigen, war aber verwirrt.

congenital defect *n*
A cleft palate is a congenital defect.

Geburtsfehler
Ein Wolfsrachen ist ein angeborener Defekt.

congestion *n*
Congestion occurs when small tubes are blocked by blood or mucus.

Stauung
Stauungen treten auf, wenn kleine Gefäße durch Blut oder Schleim blockiert sind.

conjunctivitis *n*
Conjunctivitis can be very unpleasant for the sufferer.
conjunctiva

Bindehautentzündung
Eine Bindehautentzündung kann für den Leidenden sehr unangenehm sein.
Bindehaut

consciousness *n*
I lost consciousness after the nurse gave me the second injection.

Bewusstsein
Ich wurde ohnmächtig, nachdem die Krankenschwester mir die zweite Injektion gegeben hat.

consent *v*
The patient consented reluctantly to the operation.
consent

zustimmen
Der Patient stimmte der Operation zögernd zu.
Einwilligung

constipation *n*
To avoid constipation one should eat plenty of fresh fruit and vegetables.

Verstopfung
Um Verstopfung zu meiden, soll man ausreichend frisches Obst und Gemüse essen.

consultant *n*

Konsiliararzt

In hospitals in Great Britain a consultant is a specialist who holds the highest position for a particular branch of medicine in a hospital. Outpatients also visit the consultants.

consulting hours *n*
consulting room
My GP examined me in his consulting room.

Sprechstunde
Behandlungszimmer
Mein Hausarzt untersuchte mich im Behandlungszimmer.

contact lens *n*
My brother-in-law always had trouble putting his contact lenses in.

Kontaktlinse
Mein Schwager hatte immer Probleme, seine Kontaktlinsen einzusetzen.

contagious *adj*
The isolation ward is for patients
suffering from serious illnesses which are
highly contagious.
contagious disease
contagious index

ansteckend
Die Isolierstation ist für schwerkranke
Patienten, bei denen die Ansteckungs-
gefahr sehr hoch ist.
ansteckende Krankheit
Infektionsindex

contraception *n*
contraceptive
The birthrate is lower in countries where
contraceptives are readily available.

Verhütung
Verhütungsmittel
Die Geburtenrate ist in denjenigen
Ländern niedriger, in denen Verhütungs-
mittel frei verfügbar sind.

contraction *n*
Contractions prior to childbirth are
sometimes called labour pains.

Wehe
Die Wehen vor der Geburt werden in
Englisch „labour pains" (Anstrengungs-
oder Arbeitsschmerzen) genannt.

contraindication *n*
It is safe to take this drug, provided there
are no contraindications.

Gegenanzeige
Solange keine Gegenanzeigen auftreten,
ist es ungefährlich, diese Medikamente
einzunehmen.

contrast medium *n*
A contrast medium such as barium
sulphate is used in radiography.

Kontrastmittel
Ein Kontrastmitttel, wie zum Beispiel
Bariumsulfat, wird in der Radiografie
verwendet.

contusion *n*
He had two broken ribs and contusions.

Kontusion, Prellung
Er hatte zwei gebrochene Rippen und
Prellungen.

convalescence *n*
to convalesce
He was still convalescing after his illness.

Genesung
sich von einer Krankheit erholen
Nach seiner Krankheit hatte er noch eine
Genesungszeit.

cornea *n*
A cornea transplant operation may be
necessary.

Hornhaut
Eine Hornhauttransplantation könnte
erforderlich sein.

coronary heart disease *n*
There were three cases of coronary heart
disease last week.

koronare Herzkrankheit
Es gab letzte Woche drei Fälle von
koronarer Herzkrankheit.

corpse *n*
I did not want to look at the corpse
which the police had found in the
bushes.

Leiche
Ich wollte die Leiche nicht sehen, die die
Polizei im Gebüsch gefunden hatte.

cortex *n*
The cortex cerebri is the grey matter which surrounds the cerebrum.

Cortex
Das Cortex Cerebri besteht aus den grauen Zellen, die das Cerebrum umhüllen.

cortisol *n*
Cortisol is another name for hydrocortisone, which, in its synthetic form, is used against allergies.

Cortisol
Cortisol wird in einer synthetischen Form gegen Allergien eingesetzt.

cot death *n*
The only cot death I know of was in Scotland, when I had been asked to babysit a few days earlier and had intuitively refused.

Kindstod
Der einzige mir persönlich bekannte Fall von Kindstod ereignete sich in Schottland. Man hatte mich ein paar Tage vorher darum gebeten, auf das Baby aufzupassen – intuitiv hatte ich abgelehnt.

cotton swab *n*
She cleansed the child's grazed knee with a cotton swab.

Wattebausch
Sie reinigte das aufgeschürfte Knie des Kindes mit einem Wattebausch.

cough *v*
I could not sleep, because the baby was coughing all night long.

Husten
Ich konnte nicht schlafen, weil das Baby die ganze Nacht lang hustete.

cramp *n*
My mother suffers from cramp, if she sits in the same position for too long.

Krampf
Meine Mutter leidet an Krämpfen, wenn sie zu lange in der gleichen Position sitzt.

cranium *n*
The cranium surrounds the brain.

Schädelkapsel
Die Schädelkapsel umhüllt das Gehirn.

crippled *adj*
My uncle was crippled with arthritis.

verkrüppelt
Mein Onkel war wegen Arthritis verkrüppelt.

crisis *n*
The crucial stage of a disease is referred to as the "crisis".

Krise
Die kritische Phase einer Krankheit wird „Krise" genannt.

critical *n*
His condition was critical.

kritisch
Sein Zustand war kritisch.

crush *v*
His foot had been crushed by a piece of heavy machinery.

quetschen
Sein Fuß wurde von einem schweren Gerät gequetscht.

crutch *n*
His leg was in plaster and he was walking on crutches.

Krücke
Er hatte ein Gipsbein und ging auf Krücken.

curable *n*
Many diseases which are curable today, often resulted in death in the past.

heilbar
Viele Krankheiten sind heute heilbar, die früher oft zum Tod führten.

cure *n*
Medical science is hoping to find a cure for AIDS.
cure-all

Heilung
Die Medizin hofft, ein Heilmittel gegen Aids zu entdecken.
Allheilmittel

curretage *n*
Currettage is popularly known as a D&C.

Kürettage, Ausschabung
Zu einer Ausschabung sagt man auf Englisch oft „D&C".

Cushing's disease or syndrome *n*
Cushing's disease is a result of excess corticosteroid hormones.

Cushing-Krankheit
Die Cushing-Krankheit resultiert aus einem Exzess an corticosteroiden Hormonen.

cut *n*
The boy's mother put a plaster on the cut.

Schnittwunde
Die Mutter des Jungen klebte ein Pflaster auf die Schnittwunde.

cutis *n*
"Cutis" is the technical term for "skin".

Cutis, Haut
„Cutis" ist der Fachbegriff für „Haut".

cyst *n*
Ovarian cysts are reasonably common.
cystectomy

Zyste
Eierstockzysten kommen sehr häufig vor.
Zystenausschneidung

cystitis *n*
My friend, who had cystitis, was told to drink plenty.

Blasenentzündung
Man hat meiner Freundin, die eine Blasenentzündung hatte, geraten, viel zu trinken.

D

daily dose *n*
Have you taken your daily dose of vitamins?

Tagesdosis
Hast du schon deine Tagesdosis an Vitaminen genommen?

dandruff *n*
There are special shampoos against dandruff.

Schuppen
Es gibt spezielle Shampoos gegen Schuppen.

danger *n*
He was in the intensive care unit, and we knew his life was in danger.

Gefahr
Er lag auf der Intensivstation und wir wussten, dass sein Leben in Gefahr war.

deaf *v*
My pupil is deaf in the left ear and has to wear a hearing aid.

taub
Meine Schülerin ist auf dem linken Ohr taub und muss ein Hörgerät tragen.

deaf-mute *adj*
My boyfriend's grandparents were both deaf and dumb.
deaf and dumb language

taubstumm
Die Großeltern meines Freundes waren beide taubstumm.
Taubstummensprache

death certificate *n*
When my aunt died suddenly of a heart attack, the doctor did not immediately sign the death certificate.

Totenschein
Als meine Tante plötzlich und unerwartet an einem Herzinfarkt starb, unterschrieb der Arzt nicht sofort den Totenschein.

death *n*
By forbidding drinking and driving, it has been possible to reduce the number of deaths on the roads.
deathbed

Tod
Durch das Fahrverbot nach Alkoholkonsum konnte man die Anzahl der Todesfälle auf den Straßen reduzieren.
Totenbett

decay *n*
tooth decay
Regular brushing and visits to the dentist, help prevent tooth decay.

Zerfall
Zahnfäule
Regelmäßiges Zähneputzen und Besuche beim Zahnarzt helfen, Zahnfäule zu verhindern.

decompose *v*
My neighbour died alone in her apartment and when the police finally found her, her body had started to decompose.

verwesen
Meine Nachbarin starb allein in ihrer Wohnung und als sie schließlich von der Polizei gefunden wurde, hatte ihr Körper bereits zu verwesen angefangen.

defence *n*
defence system
An allergy is an over-reaction of the body's defence system.

Abwehr
Abwehrsystem
Eine Allergie ist eine Überreaktion des Körperabwehrsystems.

deferent duct (sperm duct, deferent canal) *n*
Spermatozoa travel along the deferent duct to the urethra.

Samenleiter
Samen werden durch die Samenleiter zur Harnröhre transportiert.

deficiency *n*
deficient
Children in cold northern countries are deficient in vitamin D.

Mangelerscheinung
„mangelnd", defizient
Kindern in kalten, nördlichen Ländern fehlt Vitamin-D.

deformity *n*

Verformung, Missbildung, Verkrümmung

deformed
The physically handicapped child had a deformed leg and foot.

verformt, verkrümmt
Das körperlich behinderte Kind hatte ein verkrümmtes Bein und sein Fuß war verformt.

degeneration *n*
degenerate
Disease or injury may cause cells or tissues to degenerate.

Degeneration
degenieren
Krankheit oder Verletzungen können die Degeneration von Zellen oder Gewebe verursachen.

degree *n*
He had a temperature of 39 degrees.
The doctors were doing tests to ascertain to what degree he would be handicapped.

Grad
Er hatte 39 °C Fieber.
Die Ärzte führten Tests durch, um den Grad seiner Behinderung festzustellen.

dehydration *n*
dehydrated
When he was taken into hospital, he was dehydrated.

Dehydration
„ausgetrocknet"
Als er ins Krankenhaus eingeliefert wurde, war er fast ausgetrocknet.

delirium *n*
delirious
The patient was seriously ill and we could not speak to him, because he was delirious.

Fieberdelirium
im Delirium
Der Patient war schwerkrank und wir konnten nicht mit ihm sprechen, weil er im Delirium war.

delivery *n*
deliver
The midwife who delivered my second daughter was our neighbour.
delivery room

Entbindung
entbinden, zur Welt bringen
Die Hebamme, die meine zweite Tochter entband, war unsere Nachbarin.
Kreißsaal

delusion *n*
Psychiatric patients who are suffering from delusions cannot be persuaded by reason.

Wahn, Wahnvorstellung
Psychisch kranke Patienten, die unter Wahnvorstellungen leiden, lassen sich mit vernünftigen Argumenten nicht überzeugen.

dental assistant *n*
dental surgeon
The dental technician determined the exact shade of the crown.
dental treatment

Zahnarzthelferin
Zahnarzt
Der Zahntechniker bestimmte die genaue Farbe der Krone.
Zahnbehandlung

dentist *n*
You should visit your dentist for a check-up every six months.

Zahnarzt
Man soll alle sechs Monate zur zahnärztlichen Kontrolle gehen.

denture *n*
My mother has a full set of dentures.

Zahnprothese, Gebiss
Meine Mutter hat eine volle Zahnprothese.

Deoxyribonucleic acid *n*

Desoxyribonucleinsäure

Deoxyribonucleic acid is the full name for DNA, the substance contained in the chromosomes, responsible for the inheritance of characteristics from one's parents.

depression *n*
Depression can have a psychological or physical origin.

Depression
Die Gründe für eine Depression können psychischer oder physischer Art sein.

derma *n*
The derma, or corium, contains connective tissue, blood vessels and fat.

Derma
Das Derma oder Corium enthält Zellgewebe, Blutgefäße und Fett.

dermatitis *n*
Dermatitis is a skin condition caused by the use of aggressive cleansing products, sun exposure or allergies.

Dermatitis
Dermatitis ist eine Hautkrankheit, die durch den Gebrauch von aggressiven Reinigungsmitteln, UV-Strahlen oder Allergien verursacht werden kann.

dermatology
dermatologist
I had a rash on my left arm and made an appointment with the dermatologist.

Dermatologie
Hautarzt
Ich hatte am linken Arm einen Ausschlag und vereinbarte mit dem Hautarzt einen Termin.

desensitisation *n*
Small amounts of allergens are administered in the process of desensitisation.

Desensibilisierung
Bei der Desensibilisierung werden kleine Mengen an Allergenen verabreicht.

deteriorate *v*
His father's condition had deteriorated drastically since the last stroke.

verschlechtern
Der Zustand seines Vaters hatte sich seit dem letzten Schlaganfall drastisch verschlechtert.

development *n*
The doctors were monitoring the baby's development carefully.
develop

Entwicklung
Die Ärzte kontrollierten die Entwicklung des Babys sorgfältig.
entwickeln

de-worm *v*
Some of the children in the local kindergarten had to be de-wormed.

entwurmen
Einige Kinder im Kindergarten mussten entwurmt werden.

dextrose *n*
Dextrose occurs in the blood and tissues of animals.

Traubenzucker
Traubenzucker ist im Blut und im Gewebe von Mensch und Tier vorhanden.

diabetes mellitus *n*
Diabetes mellitus results from a lack of insulin.

Diabetes Mellitus
Diabetes Mellitus führt auf einen Mangel an Insulin zurück.

diabetic *n*

Diabetiker, an Diabetes Mellitus erkrankte Person

diagnosis *n*
It was not easy to make a diagnosis.

diagnose

Diagnose
Es war nicht einfach, zu einer Diagnose zu kommen.
diagnostizieren

dialysis *n*
Patients with malfunctioning kidneys undergo dialysis at regular intervals.

Dialyse
Patienten mit gestörter Nierenfunktion müssen sich in regelmäßigen Abständen einer Dialyse unterziehen.

diaphragm *n*
The diaphragm is a sheet of muscle located below the rib cage.

Zwerchfell
Das Zwerchfell ist eine Muskelschicht unter dem Brustkorb.

diarrhoea *n*
Diarrhoea is a typical holiday sickness in hot, humid countries with lower standards of hygiene.

Durchfall, Diarrhoe
Durchfall ist eine typische Urlaubskrankheit in warmen Ländern mit hoher Luftfeuchtigkeit und schlechten Hygienestandards.

diet *n*
She had to follow a special diet.

dietary

Diät
Sie musste sich mit einer Spezialdiät ernähren.
diätetisch

digestible *v*
digest
She had trouble sleeping, so I advised her to avoid heavy meals late at night which are difficult to digest.

digestion
digestive juice
digestive system

verdaulich
verdauen
Sie hatte Schlafstörungen, so dass ich ihr den Rat gab, vor dem Schlafengehen schwerverdauliche Mahlzeiten zu vermeiden.
Verdauung
Verdauungssaft
Verdauungstrakt

dilute *v*
One normally adds water to a substance in order to dilute it.

verdünnen
Normalerweise wird eine Substanz verdünnt, indem man Wasser hinzufügt.

diphtheria *n*
Nowadays people are vaccinated against diphtheria.

Diptherie
Heutzutage werden Leute gegen Diptherie geimpft.

disabled *adj*
He had been disabled since birth.

behindert
Er war von Geburt an behindert.

discharge *n*
There was a yellow discharge from the wound.

Ausfluss
Ein gelber Ausfluss wurde von der Wunde abgesondert.

discharge *v*
His wife was discharged from hospital.

entlassen
Seine Frau wurde aus dem Krankenhaus entlassen.

disinfection *n*
disinfect
Please disinfect the equipment after use.

Desinfektion
desinfizieren
Bitte desinfizieren Sie die Geräte nach dem Gebrauch.

dislocate *v*
I dislocated my shoulder.
dislocation

verrenken
Ich verrenkte meinen Schulter.
Verrenkung

dispensing optician *n*

A dispensing optician fits frames for glasses, but cannot prescribe lenses.

Optiker, der nicht zur Verschreibung von Linsen berechtigt ist.
Ein „Dispensing Optician" kann Brillenrahmen anpassen, aber keine Linsen verschreiben.

dissect *v*
Biologists dissect plants and animals as part of their work.

sezieren
Biologen sezieren Pflanzen und Tiere als Teil ihrer Arbeit.

dissolve *v*
Some types of aspirin dissolve in water.

auflösen
Einige Aspirinsorten lösen sich in Wasser auf.

distension *v*
An organ may be distended or enlarged.

Überdehnung
Ein Organ kann überdehnt oder vergrößert sein.

disturbed *adj*
One of the children in my class is disturbed.

verhaltensgestört
Ein Kind in meiner Klasse ist verhaltensgestört.

diuresis *n*
Diuresis refers to an excessive loss of urine.

Harnausscheidung
„Diurese" bezieht sich auf eine übermäßige Harnausscheidung.

dizziness *n*
dizzy
It was a very hot day and I had had nothing to eat; not surprisingly I felt dizzy as I stepped out of the car.

Schwindelgefühl
schwindlig
Es war ein sehr heißer Tag und ich hatte nichts gegessen, es war also keine Überraschung, dass es mir beim Aussteigen aus dem Auto schwindlig wurde.

---

domestic accident *n*
There were more injuries in casualty resulting from domestic accidents than anything else today.

Haushaltsunfall
Es gab heute mehr Verletzungen aufgrund von Haushaltsunfällen als wegen irgendwelcher anderer Ursachen.

---

donor *n*
donate
Bush asked Americans to donate blood to help the victims of the attack on the World Trade Centre towers.

Spender
spenden
Bush bat die Amerikaner, Blut zu spenden, um den Opfern des Angriffs auf die Türme des World-Trade-Centers zu helfen.

---

dosage *n*
The accuracy of the dosage is important.

Dosierung
Eine genaue Dosierung ist wichtig.

---

double chin n
Obese people often have a double chin.

Doppelkinn
Übergewichtige haben oft einen Doppelkinn.

Down's syndrome *n*

Down-Syndrom

Down's syndrome is named after the English physician, John Langdon-Down (1828-1896). A chromosome disorder is responsible for the distinctive facial features of Down's syndrome. Such children are also mentally retarded.

---

drainage *n*
drain
Pus is drained from a wound using a small tube.

Drainage
absaugen
Eiter wird aus einer Wunde abgesaugt.

---

dressing *n*
She put a clean dressing on the wound.

to apply a dressing
to change a dressing

Verband
Sie versah die Wunde mit einem sauberen Verband.
einen Verband anlegen
einen Verband wechseln

---

drip or drip-feed *n*
A drip or drip-feed is a method of administering medication to patients intravenously.

Tropf
Ein Tropf oder eine Infusion ist eine Methode, Medikamente intravenös zu verabreichen.

drown *n*
A few years ago some children drowned in the Olympic lake.

ertrinken
Vor einigen Jahren ertranken einige Kinder im Olympiasee.

drowsiness *n*
drowsy
The drugs prescribed by the GP made him feel drowsy.

Schläfrigkeit, Müdigkeit
schläfrig
Er fühlte sich durch die vom Hausarzt verschriebenen Medikamente müde.

drug *n*
drug-addict
My teacher admitted to having been a drug-addict in the past.

Droge, Arzneimittel
Drogensüchtiger
Mein Lehrer gab zu, in der Vergangenheit drogensüchtig gewesen zu sein.

dry *adj*
dry cough
I asked the chemist to give me something for a dry cough.

trocken
Reizhusten
Ich bat den Apotheker, mir etwas gegen Reizhusten zu geben.

duodenum *n*
The duodenum is the first part of the small intestine.

Duodenum, Zwölffingerdarm
Das Duodenum ist der erste Teil des Dünndarms.

dyslexia *n*

dyslexic
Dyslexic pupils often have problems with English, because it is not a phonetic language.

Lese-Rechtschreibstörung, Legasthenie, Dyslexie
Legastheniker
Legasthenische Schüler haben oft Probleme mit Englisch, weil es keine phonetische Sprache ist.

dysmenorrhoea *n*
Quite a significant percentage of women suffer from dysmenorrhoea.

Dismenorrhoe
Eine relativ große Prozentzahl von Frauen leiden unter Dismenorrhoe.

E

ear *n*
earache
I told her to go to the doctor if the earache persisted.

eardrum
earlobe

Ohr
Ohrenschmerzen
Ich empfahl ihr, zum Arzt zu gehen, sollten die Ohrenschmerzen nicht aufhören.
Trommelfell
Ohrläppchen

ear trumpet *n*
She had her ears syringed to remove the earwax.

Hörrohr
Sie ließ sich die Ohren ausspülen, um das Ohrenschmalz zu entfernen.

early *adj*
Regular check-ups make the early diagnosis of cancer possible.
early stage

früh
Regelmäßige Vorsorgeuntersuchungen ermöglichen die Frühdiagnose von Krebs.
Frühstadium

eating habit *n*
The doctor recommended that she changes her eating habits.

Essgewohnheit
Der Arzt empfahl ihr, ihre Essgewohnheiten zu ändern.

ECG – electrocardiogram *n*
An electrocardiogram is a tracing which is used to diagnose heart disease.

EKG – Elektrokardiogramm
Ein Elektrokardiogramm ist eine Aufzeichnung, die man zur Erkennung von Herzkrankheiten verwendet.

echocardiogram *n*

Echokardiogramm

echography *n*
Echography is the examination of the body using ultrasound.

Echografie
Echografie ist die Untersuchung des Körpers durch Ultraschall.

ectopic pregnancy *n*
An ectopic pregnancy occurs when the fertilised egg is situated outside the uterus.

Bauchhöhlenschwangerschaft
Bei einer Bauchhöhlenschwangerschaft befindet sich das befruchtete Ei außerhalb der Gebärmutter.

eczema *n*
Eczema patients suffer from itching and sometimes burning sensations of the affected skin.

Ekzem
Ekzempatienten leiden unter Juckreiz und manchmal einem brennenden Gefühl der betroffenen Hautpartie.

EEG – electroencephalogram *n*
An electroencephalograph produces an electroencephalogram showing the electrical impulses of the brain.

EEG – Elektroenzephalogramm
Ein Elektroenzephalograph erzeugt ein Elektroenzephalogramm, das die elektrischen Impulse des Gehirns aufzeigt.

effect *n*
The drugs were not having any effect.

Wirkung
Die Medikamente zeigten keine Wirkung.

ejaculation *n*
Ejaculation occurs during sexual intercourse.

Ejakulation
Die Ejakulation findet während des Geschlechtsverkehrs statt.

ejaculation *n*
Sexual intercourse culminates in ejaculation for the man.

Samenerguss
Der Geschlechtsverkehr endet beim Mann mit einem Samenerguss.

elbow *n*
The old lady injured her elbow when she fell down the stairs.

Ellbogen
Die alte Frau verletzte sich ihren Ellbogen, als sie die Treppe hinunterstürzte.

electrode *n*
Electrodes measure the electrical activity of the brain.

Elektrode
Elektroden messen die elektrische Aktivität des Gehirns.

electrolysis *n*
Electrolysis is used to destroy the roots of unwanted hair for cosmetic reasons.

Elektrolyse
Elektrolyse wird eingesetzt, um die Haarwurzeln aus ästhetischen Gründen zu zerstören.

electrosurgery *n*
Cauterisation is a form of electro-surgery.

Elektrochirurgie
Ausbrennung ist eine Form von Elektro-chirurgie.

elimination *n*
Urine is eliminated from the bladder.

Ausscheidung
Urin wird von der Blase ausgeschieden.

embolism *n*
When an embolus blocks a blood vessel, this is referred to as an embolism.

Embolie
Wenn ein Blutgefäß durch einen Embolus blockiert wird, wird dieser Zustand als Embolie bezeichnet.

embryo *n*
During the first three months of pregnancy, the baby is referred to as an embryo.
embryo transfer

Embryo
Während der ersten drei Monate der Schwangerschaft wird das Baby als Embryo bezeichnet.
Embryotransfer

emergency *n*
He was rushed into hospital as an emergency.
emergency call
emergency operation
emergency ward

Notfall
Er wurde als Notfall ins Krankenhaus eingeliefert.
Notruf
Notoperation
Notstation

emphysema *n*
Emphysema results from too much air in the lungs, and causes breathlessness.

Emphysem
Emphysem ist eine Folge von zu viel Luft in den Lungen und verursacht Atem-losigkeit.

emulsify *v*

emulgieren

emulsion *n*
An emulsion is a form of medicine consisting of an oily substance dispersed in another fluid.

Emulsion
Eine Emulsion ist eine Form von Medi-kament, bei der eine ölige Substanz in einer anderen Flüssigkeit aufgelöst wird.

enamel *n*
Some toothpastes can damage the enamel.

Zahnschmelz
Manche Zahnpasten können den Zahn-schmelz beschädigen.

encephalitis *n*
Encephalitis is the inflammation of the brain.

endanger *v*
I did not wish to endanger his life.

endocardiac *adj*
endocardium
The endocardium lines the heart cavities.

endoscope *n*
An endoscope is used to examine interior organs such as the stomach or bowel.

endoscopy

endure *v*
The pain was hard to endure.

enema *n*
An enema may be used to relieve the symptoms of constipation.

ENT – ear, nose and throat specialist *n*
I waited a number of weeks for an appointment with the ear, nose and throat specialist.

entry wound *n*
They discovered an entry wound in the chest of the corpse.

environmental factor *n*
Environmental factors play a role in the increase in the number of cancer patients.

enzyme *n*
Ptyalin is an enzyme contained in saliva.

epidemic *n*
There is a flu epidemic in our area at the moment.
epidemic focus

Enzephalitis
Enzephalitis nennt man die Entzündung des Gehirns.

gefährden
Ich hatte nicht die Absicht, sein Leben zu gefährden.

endokardial
Endokardium
Das Endokardium bildet die Innenseite der Herzkammer.

Endoskop
Ein Endoskop wird zur Untersuchung innerer Organe wie Magen und Darm verwendet.
Endoskopie

ertragen
Der Schmerz war schwer zu ertragen.

Einlauf
Ein Einlauf wird angewandt, um Verstopfung zu lindern.

Hals-Nasen-Ohren-Arzt

Ich wartete einige Wochen lang auf einen Termin beim Hals-Nasen-Ohren-Arzt.

Eintrittswunde, Einschuss
Die Leiche wies eine Einschusswunde in der Brust auf.

Umwelteinfluss
Umwelteinflüsse spielen eine Rolle bei der numerischen Zunahme von Krebspatienten.

Enzym
Ptylin ist ein im Speichel enthaltenes Enzym.

Epidemie
Momentan gibt es eine Grippeepidemie in unserer Gegend.
epidemischer Herd

epidermis *n*
The epidermis is the outer layer of the skin.

Epidermis
Die Epidermis ist die äußere Hautschicht.

epididymis *n*
Sperm are stored in the epididymes.

Nebenhoden
Sperma wird in den Nebenhoden gespeichert.

epidural anaesthetic *n*
My friend was given an epidural anaesthetic when her baby was delivered, and was able to witness the birth.

Epiduralanästhesie
Meine Freundin bekam eine Epiduralanästhesie bei der Entbindung und konnte so die Geburt miterleben.

epilepsy *n*
epileptic
My uncle was an epileptic and always had to take medication to prevent fits.

Epilepsie
Epileptiker
Mein Onkel war Epileptiker und musste immer Medikamente nehmen, um Anfälle zu vermeiden.

equipment *n*
Some hospitals in the third world are badly in need of new equipment.

Ausstattung, Geräte
Manche Krankenhäuser in der dritten Welt benötigen dringend eine neue Ausstattung.

erection *n*
Failure to have an erection may be due to physical or psychological causes.

Erektion
Der Ausfall einer Erektion kann physische oder psychische Ursachen haben.

Eustachian tube *n*
The Eustachian tube equalises pressure in the eardrum.

Eustachische Röhre
Die Eustachische Röhre gleicht den Druck im Trommelfell aus.

euthanasia *n*
I am sure euthanasia will be possible for my generation.

Euthanasie
Ich glaube, dass Euthanasie in meiner Generation möglich sein wird.

evacuation *n*
evacuate
They gave him an enema to evacuate his bowels.

Evakuation, Entleerung
entleeren
Sie machten einen Einlauf, um den Darm zu entleeren.

examine *v*
He asked the doctor to examine his left ankle.

untersuchen
Er bat den Arzt, sein linkes Fußgelenk zu untersuchen.

excretion *n*
excrete
Body waste should be excreted at regular intervals.

Ausscheidung
ausscheiden
Körperabfallprodukte sollen regelmäßig ausgeschieden werden.

exhaustion *n*
He had been working too hard and was exhibiting symptoms of exhaustion.

Erschöpfung
Er hatte zu hart gearbeitet und es zeigten sich Symptome der Erschöpfung.

expectant *adj*
The man offered his seat in the waiting room to the expectant mother.

schwanger
Der Mann bot der Schwangeren im Wartezimmer seinen Stuhl an.

expire *v*
To expire is to breathe out.

ausatmen
Das englische Wort „expire" heißt „ausatmen".

extraction *n*
Unfortunately the dentist had to extract the tooth.

Herauslösen, Extrahieren
Leider musste der Zahnarzt den Zahn ziehen.

F

facial *adj*
I could see from his facial expression that he was not happy with the treatment.

fazial
Ich konnte an seinem Gesichtsausdruck erkennen, dass er mit der Behandlung nicht zufrieden war.

faeces n pl
Faeces are excreted from the intestines.

Fäzes, Stuhl
Der Stuhl wird vom Darm ausgeschieden.

faint *v*
It was very hot in the theatre and she fainted during the interval.

ohnmächtig werden
Es war sehr heiß im Theater und sie wurde während der Pause ohnmächtig.

fallopian tube *n*
If the fallopian tubes are blocked, then a pregnancy is not possible.
fallopian tube pregnancy

Eileiter
Wenn die Eileiter blockiert sind, ist eine Schwangerschaft nicht möglich.
Eileiterschwangerschaft

false pains *n*
She thought she was in labour, but they were false pains.

Vorwehen
Sie dachte, sie bekäme Wehen, es waren aber Vorwehen.

family background *n*
The psychologist was interested in her family background.

Familienhintergrund
Der Psychologe interessierte sich für ihren Familienhintergrund.

family therapy *n*
Family therapy is a form of psychotherapy which has the aim of improving family relationships.

Familientherapie
Familientherapie ist eine Form der Psychotherapie, die das Ziel hat, Beziehungen in der Familie zu verbessern.

fango *n*
fangopack
*Fangopacks relieve the symptoms of
rheumatism and arthritis.*

Fango
Fangopackung
*Fangopackungen lindern die Symptome
von Rheuma und Arthritis.*

farsightedness *n*
Farsightedness increases with age.

Weitsichtigkeit
*Weitsichtigkeit schreitet mit dem Alter
fort.*

fasting *n*
*Fasting is an extremely drastic way of
losing weight.*

Fasten, Nulldiät
*Fasten ist eine extreme Methode
abzunehmen.*

fat *adj*
*We usually say "overweight" rather than
"fat".*

dick
*Wir sprechen normalerweise von „Über-
gewicht" und bezeichnen Leute nicht als
„dick".*

fat *n*
*One should avoid too much fat in one's
diet.*
fatty acid
fatty liver
fatty metamorphosis of liver

Fett
*Man soll beim Essen zu viel Fett ver-
meiden.*
Fettsäure
Fettleber
Leberverfettung

fatal *adj*
The car crash was fatal.

tödlich
Der Autounfall war tödlich.

fatherhood *n*
*The doctors did tests to prove
fatherhood.*

Vaterschaft
*Die Ärzte führten Tests durch, um die
Vaterschaft nachzuweisen.*

fatigue *n*
*The bus driver fell asleep at the wheel,
due to fatigue.*
fatigue fracture

Müdigkeit
*Der Busfahrer schlief wegen Müdigkeit
am Lenkrad ein.*
Ermüdungsfraktur

fear of heights *n*
*I never go climbing and I don't like tall
buildings because of my fear of heights.*

Höhenangst
*Aufgrund meiner Höhenangst gehe ich
nie Bergsteigen und ich mag auch keine
hohen Gebäude.*

fee *n*
*The doctor's fee for a relatively simple
examination was exorbitant.*

Gebühr, Honorar
*Das Ärztehonorar war für eine relativ
einfache Untersuchung überhöht.*

feeble *adj*
*The patient was still feeble after the
operation.*

kraftlos, schwach
*Der Patient war nach der Operation noch
schwach.*

feeding bottle *n*
The baby sucked a little bit, screwed up his face and threw the feeding bottle onto the ground.

Saugflasche
Das Baby saugte ein wenig, machte ein komisches Gesicht und warf die Saugflasche auf den Boden.

female complaint *n*
Osteoporosis is a typical female complaint due to lack of oestrogen after the menopause.

Frauenleiden
Osteoporose ist aufgrund Östrogenmangels nach den Wechseljahren ein typisches Frauenleiden.

femur *n*
The man had fractured his femur.

femoral neck vein

Oberschenkel
Der Mann hatte sich seinen Oberschenkel gebrochen.
Oberschenkelvene

fertile *adj*
fertility
Women who take fertility drugs often have multiple births.

fruchtbar
Fruchtbarkeit
Fruchtbarkeitsfördernde Medikamente verursachen oft Mehrfachgeburten.

fester *v*
The child had hurt his knee and the wound was beginning to fester.

eitern
Das Kind verletzte sich das Knie und die Wunde begann zu eitern.

fever *n*
Many illnesses are accompanied by a fever.

Fieber
Fieber ist ein Begleitsymptom vieler Krankheiten.

fibrosis *n*
Fibrosis is caused by inflammation.

fibrositis

Fibrose
Fibrose ist auf eine Entzündung zurückzuführen.
Fibrositis

fibula *n*
The fibula is one of the two bones below the knee.

Wadenbein
Das Wadenbein ist einer der beiden Knochen unter dem Knie.

filling *n*
The dentist replaced three fillings for me yesterday.

Plombe, Füllung
Der Zahnarzt ersetzte mir gestern drei Füllungen.

finger pad *n*
fingerprint
Forensic scientists examined the book for fingerprints.

Fingerkuppe
Fingerabdruck
Gerichtsmediziner untersuchten das Buch nach Fingerabdrücken.

first aid *n*
The Red Cross offers first aid courses.

Erste Hilfe
Das Rote Kreuz bietet Erste-Hilfe-Kurse an.

fissure *n*
Fissures divide organs into lobes.

Schrunde, Fissur
Schrunden teilen Organe in Lappen ein.

flabby *adj*
The skin at the backs of her thighs was very flabby and unsightly.

schlaff
Die Haut an ihren Oberschenkeln war sehr schlaff und sah nicht schön aus.

flatulence *n*
Certain food products are prone to causing flatulence.

Blähungen
Bestimmte Lebensmittel fördern Blähungen.

flea *n*
Pets whose fur is infested with fleas should be treated.

Floh
Flohbefallene Haustiere sollten behandelt werden.

flesh wound *n*
The bullet luckily only caused a flesh wound.

Fleischwunde
Die Kugel verursachte glücklicherweise nur eine Fleischwunde.

fluid balance *n*
It is important to maintain the body fluid balance.

Flüssigkeitshaushalt
Es ist wichtig, den Flüssigkeitshaushalt des Körpers zu erhalten.

foetus *n*

Fötus

After conception the fertilised ovum is referred to as an embryo. In the second or third month of pregnancy the embryo becomes a fetus, or **foetus**, when it possesses the distinctive features of a human baby, or in the case of animals, of the mature species.

**foetus monitoring
foetus wastage**

**Fötusüberwachung
künstlicher Abort**

fontanelle *n*
The fontanelle is the soft spot in the skull of an infant.

Fontanelle
Die Fontanelle ist der weiche Punkt im Schädel eines Babys oder Kleinkindes.

food poisoning *n*
My cousin was taken into hospital with food poisoning after eating fish during his holiday.

Lebensmittelvergiftung
Mein Cousin wurde mit einer Lebensmittelvergiftung ins Krankenhaus eingeliefert, nachdem er im Urlaub Fisch gegessen hatte.

forceps *n*
My first daughter was delivered with forceps.
**forceps delivery
forceps extraction**

Zange
Meine erste Tochter war eine Zangengeburt.
**Zangengeburt
Zangenextraktion**

forearm *n*
The patient had a severe burn on the forearm.

Unterarm
Der Patient hatte eine schwere Brandwunde am Unterarm.

forensic medicine *n*
Forensic medicine is the branch of medicine which produces medical evidence for the courts.

Gerichtsmedizin
Die Gerichtsmedizin ist ein Arbeitsbereich, der dem Gericht medizinische Beweise liefert.

frontal *adj*
frontal baldness
frontal headache
frontal mirror
frontal region

Stirn-
Stirnglatze
Stirnkopfschmerz
Stirnspiegel
Stirnregion

fungal infection *n*
Fungal infections can affect various parts of the body.

Pilzerkrankung
Pilzerkrankungen können verschiedene Körperteile angreifen.

further treatment *n*
No further treatment is necessary.

Weiterbehandlung
Es ist keine Weiterbehandlung notwendig.

G

gall bladder *n*
gall stones
The patient was admitted to hospital with suspected gall stones.

Gallenblase
Gallensteine
Der Patient wurde mit Verdacht auf Gallensteine ins Krankenhaus eingeliefert.

gap *n*
The child had lost several milk teeth, and the gaps were visible when he smiled.

Zahnlücke
Das Kind hatte einige Milchzähne verloren und wenn es lächelte, konnte man die Lücken sehen.

gargle *v*
When I had a sore throat as a child, my mother made me gargle.

gurgeln
Wenn ich als Kind Halsweh hatte, sorgte meine Mutter immer dafür, dass ich gurgelte.

gasp *v*
The man was overweight and out of condition – he was gasping for breath as he reached the top of the stairs.
to gasp for breath
gasp

japsen, nach Luft schnappen
Der Mann hatte Übergewicht und keine Kondition – er schnappte nach Luft, als er die oberste Treppe erreichte.
nach Luft schnappen
schweres Atmen

gastric acid *n*
Too much gastric acid can attack the lining of the stomach.
gastric juice
gastric lavage
gastric ulcer

Magensäure
Ein Übermaß an Magensäure kann die Magenschleimhaut angreifen.
Magensaft
Magenspülung
Magengeschwür

gastritis *n*
An upset stomach is the false popular term for gastritis.

Magenschleimhautentzündung
In der Umgangssprache bezeichnet man Gastritis fälschlicherweise als eine „Magenverstimmung".

gastroscopy *n*
The patient had been complaining of serious stomach pains and so the doctors decided to perform a gastroscopy.

Magenspiegelung
Der Patient klagte über ernsthafte Magenschmerzen, so dass die Ärzte sich entschieden, eine Magenspiegelung durchzuführen.

gauze *n*
The nurse bandaged the child's ankle with a gauze bandage.

gauze bandage
gauze pad
gauze strap

Verbandmull
Die Krankenschwester verband das Fußgelenk des Kindes mit einer Mullbinde.
Mullbinde
Tupfer
Gazestreifen

gemellology *n*
The professor was engaged in gemellology.

Zwillingsforschung
Der Professor arbeitete an der Zwillingsforschung.

general condition *n*
His general condition was poor due to excessive alcohol consumption and smoking.
general medicine

allgemeines Befinden
Sein allgemeines Befinden war aufgrund übermäßigen Alkoholkonsums und Rauchens schlecht.
Allgemeinmedizin

general practitioner

Allgemeinarzt

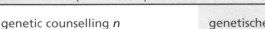
The British National Health Service has a system whereby patients are registered with a **general practitioner**. This doctor then provides them with a transfer to a specialist, as the need arises. The lengthy waiting lists for such appointments are well known and often a reason for patients to seek private treatment.

genetic counselling *n*
Couples wishing to have a child with hereditary diseases in the family, may wish to attend genetic counselling.

genetische Beratung
Paare, die sich ein Kind wünschen und vererbbare Krankheiten in der Familie haben, konsultieren möglicherweise genetische Beratung.

genetic engineering *n*
*Genetic engineering is a very
controversial topic.*

Gentechnologie
*Gentechnologie ist ein kontrovers
diskutiertes Thema.*

genital *adj*
*It can be embarrassing to have to
describe symptoms in the genital area to
the doctor.*
genital zone
genital organ

genital
*Es kann peinlich sein, dem Arzt
Symptome in Genitalbereich zu
beschreiben.*
Genitalbereich
Genitalorgan

geriatrics *n*
geriatric
*She visited her seventy-year old mother
while she was in the geriatric ward.*

Geriatrie
geriatrisch
*Sie besuchte ihre siebzigjährige Mutter,
während sie auf der geriatrischen Station
war.*

germ *n*
*She disinfected the surfaces in order to
ensure a germ-free environment.*

Keim
*Sie desinfizierte die Oberflächen um eine
keimfreie Umgebung sicherzustellen.*

German measles *n*
*My aunt had German measles when she
was a child.*

Röteln
Meine Tante hatte als Kind Röteln.

germicide *n*
*A germicide kills pathogenic
microorganisms.*

Germizid
*Ein Germizid tötet pathogenische
Mikroorganismen.*

gerontology *n*
*Gerontology is the study of the aging
process.*

Gerontologie
*Gerontologie ist die Wissenschaft des
Alterns.*

gingivitis *n*
*Gingivitis is the technical term for
inflammation of the gums.*

Zahnfleischentzündung
*„Gingivitis" ist in England der technische
Begriff für eine Zahnfleischentzündung.*

gland *n*
*A gland is an organ which synthesises
and secretes substances required by the
body.*

Drüse
*Eine Drüse ist ein Organ, das Substanzen,
die der Körper braucht, synthetisiert und
absondert.*

glasses *n*
*My cousin was extremely short-sighted
and needed glasses.*

Brille
*Mein Cousine war extrem kurzsichtig und
brauchte eine Brille.*

glaucoma *n*
*Glaucoma is a serious disease of
the eye.*

Glaukom
*Ein Glaukom ist eine ernsthafte Augen-
krankheit.*

glucose *n*
Glucose is an endogenous source of energy.

Glukose
Glukose ist eine körpereigene Energiequelle.

gonorrhoea *n*
Gonorrhoea is an infectious, sexually-transmitted disease.

Tripper
Tripper gilt als eine ansteckende, sexuell übertragbare Krankheit.

goose pimples n pl
People get goose pimples when they feel cold.

Gänsehaut
Menschen bekommen eine Gänsehaut, wenn ihnen kalt ist.

gout *n*
A symptom of gout is pain in the big toe caused by deposits of sodium urate.

Gicht
Ein Symptom der Gicht sind durch Ablagerungen verursachte Schmerzen im großen Zeh.

grasp reflex *n*
The grasp reflex causes newborn babies to close their hands tightly around, for example, their mother's fingers.

Greifreflex
Der Greifreflex sorgt dafür, dass neugeborene Babies ihre Hände fest um die Finger der Mutter schließen.

graze *v*
Small children often fall over and graze their knees.

abschürfen
Kleinkinder fallen oft hin und schürfen sich die Knie ab.

grief *n*
Grief can have an effect on the psychological well-being of the person.

Trauer
Trauer kann eine Auswirkung auf das psychische Wohlbefinden des Menschen haben.

groin *n*
Describing in actual fact the join between the legs and abdomen, the word "groin" is sometimes used euphemistically to refer to the genitals.

Leiste
Das englische Wort „groin" ist eigentlich die Verbindung zwischen Bein und Abdomen, wird aber manchmal euphemistisch für die Genitalien genommen.

group practice *n*
Group practices have the advantage that doctors can share surgery hours.

Gemeinschaftspraxis
Gemeinschaftspraxen haben den Vorteil, dass Ärzte sich die Sprechstunden einteilen können.

growth *n*
growth hormone

Wachstum, Tumor
Wachstumshormon

Growth is the normal development in size of a child. A growth is the abnormal development of tissue, such as that which constitutes a tumour.

gunshot wound *n*
The armed bank robber attempted to make a getaway, but he was too slow due to a gunshot wound in the shoulder, and the police caught him.

Schussverletzung
Der bewaffnete Bankräuber versuchte zu entkommen, aber er war aufgrund einer Schussverletzung in der Schulter zu langsam und die Polizei nahm ihn fest.

gynaecologist *n*
The gynaecologist prescribed the pill.

Gynäkologe
Der Gynäkologe verschrieb die Antibabypille.

haematoma *n*
A haemotoma is a blood clot in an organ or tissue which is caused by a break in the wall of a blood vessel.

Hämatom
Ein Hämatom ist die Blutgerinnung in einem Organ oder Gewebe, die durch das Eindringen durch die Außenschicht eines Blutgefäßes verursacht wird.

haemoglobin *n*
Haemoglobin gives blood its red colour and transports oxygen.
to test for haemoglobin

Hämoglobin, Hb
Hämoglobin gibt dem Blut die rote Farbe und transportiert Sauerstoff.
den Hb-Gehalt bestimmen

haemophilia *n*
Some haemophilia patients were given blood transfusions with infected blood.
haemophiliac

Bluterkrankheit
Einigen Patienten wurden Bluttransfusionen mit infiziertem Blut gegeben.
Bluter

haemorrhoids n pl
Haemorrhoids may, or may not, need surgical treatment.

Hämorrhoiden
Hämorrhoiden benötigen manchmal chirurgische Behandlung.

hairloss *n*
Men sometimes suffer from hairloss resulting in baldness, when they are quite young.

Haarausfall
Männer leiden oft an Haarausfall, der zur Kahlheit führt, auch wenn sie jung sind.

hallucinate *v*
hallucination
Drugs such as LSD cause hallucinations.

hallucinogenic

halluzinieren
Halluzination
Drogen wie LSD bewirken Halluzinationen.
halluzinogen

handicap *n*
handicapped
I have two physically handicapped participants in my English class.

Behinderung
behindert
Ich habe zwei körperbehinderte Teilnehmer in meiner Englischklasse.

harden v
hardening
In layman's terms we say "hardening of the arteries" for arteriosclerosis.

verhärten
Verhärtung
In der Laiensprache reden wir von einer Verhärtung der Arterien anstatt von Arteriosclerose.

harelip n
A harelip is a birth defect.

Hasenscharte
Eine Hasenscharte ist ein Geburtsfehler.

harmful adj
Some household products may contain chemical substances which are harmful.

harmful to health
harmless

schädlich
Manche Haushaltsprodukte können schädliche chemische Substanzen enthalten.
gesundheitsschädlich
ungefährlich

have a baby v
The couple wanted desperately to have a baby.

Kinderkriegen
Das Paar wollte unbedingt ein Kind bekommen.

hay fever n
My son gets hay fever every year.

Heuschnupfen
Mein Sohn bekommt jedes Jahr Heuschnupfen.

head n
headache
head bandage
head birth
She took an aspirin, because she had a headache.
to hit the head

Kopf
Kopfschmerzen
Kopfverband
Kopflage
Sie nahm eine Aspirin, weil sie Kopfschmerzen hatte.
sich den Kopf stoßen

heal v
The cut was healing nicely.
healed
health n
health care
Private health care is expensive.
health insurance
health profession
healthy

heilen
Die Schnittwunde heilte schön.
verheilt
Gesundheit
Gesundheitswesen
Private Gesundheitsfürsorge ist teuer.
Krankenversicherung
Heilberuf
gesund

hear v
hearing
The elderly gentlemen was hard of hearing.
hearing acuity
hearing aid
to lose hearing

hören
Gehör, Gehörsinn
Der ältere Herr war schwerhörig.

Hörschärfe
Hörapparat
das Gehör verlieren

heart *n*
heart attack
heart beat
heartburn
I occasionally suffered from heartburn when I was pregnant.
heart complaint
heart disease
heart failure
heart hurry

heart-lung-machine *n*
After the accident the man was attached to a heart-lung-machine, which was keeping him alive. Then family had to decide whether to have the machine switched off.
heartrate
heart valve
heart valve prosthesis

heat *n*
heat exhaustion
heat spot
heat stroke
It was a very hot, sunny day,and several patients were admitted to hospital with heatstroke.

heel *n*
The chiropodist removed the hard skin from the woman's heels.
heelbone
heelspur

help *n*
The woman was crying for help, when the emergency services found her trapped in the garage.

hepatitis *n*
The man contracted hepatitis when he was on holiday in Africa.

herb *n*
herbal medicine
Herbal medicine is a natural alternative to conventional western medicine.

Herz
Herzinfarkt
Herzschlag
Sodbrennen
Ich litt während der Schwangerschaft gelegentlich an Sodbrennen.
Herzbeschwerden
Herzkrankheit
Herzversagen
Herzrasen

Herz-Lungen-Maschine
Nach dem Unfall wurde der Mann an eine Herz-Lungen-Maschine angeschlossen, die ihn am Leben erhielt. Nun musste sich seine Familie entscheiden, ob man die Maschine ausschalteten sollte.
Herzfrequenz
Herzklappe
Herzklappenprothese

Hitze
Hitzekollaps
Hitzepickel
Hitzschlag
Es war ein sehr warmer, sonniger Tag und einige Patienten wurden mit Hitzschlag ins Krankenhaus eingeliefert.

Ferse
Der Fußpfleger entfernte die Hornhaut an den Fersen der Patientin.
Fersenbein
Fersensporn

Hilfe
Die Frau schrie nach Hilfe, als der Notdienst sie in der Garage eingeschlossen fand.

Hepatitis
Der Mann erkrankte an Hepatitis, als er in Afrika im Urlaub war.

Kraut
Kräutermedizin, Kräuterheilkunde
Kräuterheilkunde gilt als eine natürliche Alternative zur konventionellen westlichen Medizin.

hereditary *adj*
Some diseases are hereditary.
hereditary factor
hereditary transmission

vererbbar
Manche Krankheiten sind vererbbar.
Erbanlage
Vererbung

herpes *n*
Herpes is extremely contagious.

Herpes
Herpes ist extrem ansteckend.

heterosexuality *n*
Heterosexuality is the attraction to the opposite sex.

Heterosexualität
Heterosexualität ist die Eigenschaft, sich vom anderen Geschlecht angezogen zu fühlen.

hiccough *n*
Folk medicine had several remedies for the treatment of hiccoughs, such as dropping a penny down one's back.

Schluckauf
Die Volksmedizin hatte einige Heilmethoden für die Behandlung von Schluckauf, so auch eine Münze zwischen Kleidung und Rücken herunterrutschen lassen.

high risk delivery *n*
Since my second daughter was a high risk delivery, the doctor wanted me to have her in the county hospital.

Risikogeburt
Weil meine zweite Tochter eine Risikogeburt war, wollte der Arzt, dass ich sie im Kreiskrankenhaus bekäme.

hinge joint *n*
The joint between the upper and lower arm is a hinge joint.

Scharniergelenk
Das Gelenk zwischen Ober- und Unterarm ist ein Scharniergelenk.

hip *n*
"Hip" is sometimes used as an abbreviation of "hip joint", a joint which the elderly sometimes need to have replaced.
hip replacement surgery

Hüfte
Das englische Wort „hip" wird manchmal als Abkürzung für das Hüftgelenk verwendet, ein Gelenk, das bei älteren Menschen manchmal ersetzt werden muss.
Hüftenersatzchirurgie

Hippocratic oath *n*
Doctors swear the Hippocratic oath before practising medicine.

Eid des Hippokrates
Ärzte schwören den Eid des Hippokrates, bevor sie anfangen zu praktizieren.

histamine *n*
When the body is confronted with a substance to which it is allergic, it reacts by producing histamines.

Histamin
Wenn der Körper mit einer Substanz konfrontiert wird, auf die er mit einer Allergie reagiert, werden im Körper Histamine erzeugt.

HIV positive *adj*
HIV test
HIV tests are being carried out in Africa.

HIV-positiv
HIV-Test
Viele HIV-Tests werden in Afrika durchgeführt.

hoarse *adj*
hoarseness
If I have to teach in a large, cold room, I often suffer with hoarseness the next day.

holistic *adj*
Holistic medicine does not restrict itself to treating the symptoms of the disease, but treats the patient as an entire entity.

hollow of the knee *n*
He had a sharp pain in the hollow of his knee.

homeopathy *n*
homeopathic
Homeopathic medicines are very popular.

homosexuality *n*
Homosexuality is the attraction to sexual partners of the same sex.

homosexual

hormone *n*
hormone deficiency
Hormone deficiency can be treated by the administration of hormones.

hormone replacement therapy *n*
HRT, or hormone replacement therapy, is the administration of hormones to alleviate the symptoms of the menopause.

hospital *n*
London has a number of famous teaching hospitals.

hot *adj*
hot flushes
Hot flushes are a symptom of the menopause.
hot water bottle

heiser
Heiserkeit
Wenn ich in einem großen, kalten Raum unterrichten muss, leide ich am nächsten Tag oft unter Heiserkeit.

ganzheitlich
Ganzheitliche Medizin begrenzt sich nicht alleine darauf, Krankheitssymptome zu behandeln, sondern sie sieht den Patienten als ganzes Wesen.

Kniekehle
Er hatte gestern einen stechenden Schmerz in der Kniekehle.

Homöopathie
homöopathisch
Homöopathische Heilmittel sind sehr beliebt.

Homosexualität
Homosexualität ist die Eigenschaft, sich zu sexuellen Partnern des gleichen Geschlechts hingezogen zu fühlen.
homosexuell

Hormon
Hormonmangel
Hormonmangel kann durch die Verabreichung von Hormonen ausgeglichen werden.

Hormonersatztherapie
Eine Hormonersatztherapie ist die Verabreichung von Hormonen, um die Symptome der Wechseljahre zu lindern.

Krankenhaus
In London befinden sich einige berühmte Krankenhäuser, in denen Ärzte ausgebildet werden.

heiß
Hitzewallungen
Hitzewallungen sind ein Symptom der Wechseljahre.
Wärmflasche

house dust allergy *n*
People with a house dust allergy have to vacuum their rooms carefully and regularly.

Hausstauballergie
Leute mit einer Hausstauballergie müssen ihre Zimmer sorgfältig und regelmäßig saugen.

household remedy *n*
My grandmother knew a lot of household remedies, such butter for bruises.

Hausmittel
Meine Großmutter kannte viele Hausmittel, wie zum Beispiel Butter gegen Prellungen.

hydrocephalus *n*
Babies with hydrocephalus have to be monitored very carefully.

Wasserkopf
Babys mit einem Wasserkopf müssen sehr sorgfältig überwacht werden.

hydrogen *n*
Hydrogen is one of the constituents of water.
hydrogen-ion concentration

Wasserstoff
Wasserstoff ist in Wasser enthalten.

Wasserstoffionenkonzentration

hygiene *n*
hygienic
Disposible items are often used, because they are hygienic.

Hygiene
hygienisch
Wegwerfartikel werden oft verwendet, weil sie hygienisch sind.

hymen *n*
hymen atresia
hymenitis

Jungfernhäutchen
Hymenverschluss
Hymenentzündung

hypersensitive *adj*
If someone is hypersensitive to something, this may have psychological causes.

überempfindlich
Wenn jemand überempfindlich auf etwas reagiert, könnte dies eventuell psychische Ursachen haben.

hypertension *n*
Hypertension sufferers may have to take medication.

Bluthochdruck
Leute, die an Bluthochdruck leiden, müssen manchmal Medikamente nehmen.

hypnosis *n*

Hypnosis is used in psychology.

hypnotherapy
hypnotise

Hypnose, künstlicher Teilschlaf
Hypnose wird in der Psychologie verwendet.
Hypnosebehandlung
hypnotisieren

hypotension *n*
People with hypotension are said to live longer.
hypotensive

niedriger Blutdruck
Angeblich leben Leute mit niedrigem Blutdruck länger.
Unterdruck-

hypothermia *n*
*One sometimes reads in English
newspapers of old people dying of
hypothermia, because they cannot afford
the heating.
Last year senior citizens were granted a
heating allowance.*

Hypothermie
*Man liest manchmal in den englischen
Zeitungen über alte Leute, die an
Hypothermie sterben, weil sie sich die
Heizkosten nicht leisten können.
Letztes Jahr bekamen Senioren einen
Zuschuss für Heizung.*

hysterectomy *n*
*Hysterectomies are sometimes performed
on women who suffer from extremely
heavy periods.*

Gebärmutterentfernung
*Eine Gebärmutterentfernung wird manch-
mal bei Frauen durchgeführt, die an extrem starken Monatsblutungen leiden.*

hysteria *n*
*The traditional cure for hysteria was a
slap on the cheek!*

Hysterie
*Das traditionelle Heilmittel gegen
Hysterie war ein Klaps auf die Wange.*

icebag *n*
*He put an icebag on the bruise, which
made him feel a little better.*

Eisbeutel
*Er legte einen Eisbeutel auf die Prellung,
wonach es ihm etwas besser ging.*

ideal weight *n*
*She was hoping to lose a few kilos and
regain her ideal weight.*

Idealgewicht
*Sie hoffte, ein paar Kilo abzunehmen, um
ihr Idealgewicht zurückzugewinnen.*

illegitimate *adj*
*The little boy was illegitimate and, in
fact, no-one knew who his father was.*

unehelich
*Der kleine Junge war unehelich und nie-
mand wusste, wer eigentlich sein Vater
war.*

illness *n*
*He had just returned to work after a
serious illness.*

Krankheit
*Er hat nach einer schweren Krankheit die
Arbeit wieder aufgenommen.*

immune *adj*
  immune body
  immune cell
  immune system
*He had been ill for a long time and his
immune system had been weakened.*

immun
  Antikörper
  Immunzelle
  Immunsystem
*Er war lange Zeit krank gewesen und sein
Immunsystem war geschwächt.*

immunity *n*
  to acquire immunity
  immunization
  immunology

Immunität
  Immunität erlangen
  Immunisierung
  Immunitätslehre

implant *n*
The body may reject implants.

Implantat
*Bei Implantaten kann es zu einer Ab-
wehrreaktion des Körpers kommen.*

impotence *n*
impotent
*If a man is impotent, his wife can still
have a baby by artificial insemination.*

Impotenz
impotent
*Wenn ein Mann impotent ist, kann seine
Frau dennoch ein Baby durch künstliche
Befruchtung bekommen.*

in vitro *adj*
*In vitro fertilisation makes it possible for
some women to have a baby, who other-
wise could not.*

im Reagenzglas
*Eine Befruchtung im Reagenzglas macht
es einigen Frauen möglich, Kinder zu
bekommen, die sonst nicht dazu in der
Lage wären.*

incest *n*
*Incest should be avoided because of the
dangers of hereditary diseases.*

Inzest
*Inzest soll wegen der Gefahr vererbbarer
Krankheiten vermieden werden.*

incinerator *n*
*Hospital waste is put in the incinerator to
prevent the spread of germs.*

Verbrennungsofen
*Krankenhausabfälle kommen in einen
Verbrennungsofen, um die Verbreitung
von Keimen auszuschließen.*

incision *n*
*The surgeon made an incision in the
patient's abdomen.*

Einschnitt
*Der Chirurg machte einen Schnitt in den
Bauch des Mannes.*

incisor *n*
*He had to have one of his upper incisors
crowned.*

Schneidezahn
*Auf einen seiner oberen Schneidezähne
musste eine Krone aufgesetzt werden.*

incoherent *n*
*The patient was under sedation and,
although she tried to speak, was
incoherent.*

unverständlich, inkohärent
*Die Patientin wurde betäubt und, obwohl
sie zu sprechen versuchte, konnte man sie
nicht verstehen.*

incompatible *n*
*The two blood groups were
incompatible.*

inkompatibel, unverträglich
*Die zwei Blutgruppen waren in-
kompatibel.*

incontinence *n*
*The very elderly sometimes suffer from
incontinence.*

Inkontinenz
*Sehr alte Leute leiden manchmal an
Inkontinenz.*

incubation period *n*
*The incubation period for measles is
about two weeks.*

Inkubationszeit
*Die Inkubationszeit bei Masern beträgt
circa zwei Wochen.*

incubator *n*
*Newborn babies are put into an
incubator, when they need oxygen.*

incubator care

Brutkasten
*Neugeborene Babys kommen in einen
Brutkasten, wenn sie Sauerstoff be-
nötigen.*
Inkubatorpflege

incurable *adj*
*Some diseases which used to be incurable
can nowadays be treated effectively.*

incurability

unheilbar
*Einige Krankheiten, die früher unheilbar
waren, können heutzutage wirksam
behandelt werden.*
Unheilbarkeit

index finger *n*
*We use our index finger when we want
to point to something.*

Zeigefinger
*Wir verwenden unsere Zeigefinger, wenn
wir auf etwas zeigen wollen.*

indigestible *adj*
Spicy food can be rather indigestible.

unverdaulich
*Scharfes Essen kann ziemlich unverdau-
lich sein.*

indigestion *n*
*He always had indigestion after eating
fish and chips.*

Verdauungsstörung
*Er hatte immer Verdauungsstörungen,
nachdem er „Fish und Chips" gegessen
hatte.*

induce *v*
induce anaesthesia
induce pain

auslösen, einleiten
die Narkose einleiten
Schmerzen verursachen

industrial accident *n*
*He received compensation, because his
foot injury was an industrial accident.*

Betriebsunfall
*Er erhielt Schadensersatz, weil die
Fußverletzung ein Betriebsunfall war.*

inebriated *adj*
*A polite way of saying someone is drunk
is to say that he or she is inebriated.*

im Rausch, betrunken
*Das englische Adjektiv „inebriated" ist
eine höfliche Art zu sagen, dass jemand
betrunken ist.*

infancy *n*
*The singer had been talented since his
infancy.*

Kleinkindalter
*Der Sänger war seit dem Kleinkindalter
talentiert.*

infant *n*
infant death

Säugling, Kleinkind
Säuglingstod

infant formula *n*
*The mother ceased breast-feeding when
her son was six months old and gave him
infant formula.*

Milchfertignahrung
*Die Mutter hörte auf zu stillen, als ihr
Sohn sechs Monate alt war und gab ihm
Milchfertignahrung.*

infantilism *n*
Infantilism is a psychological condition whereby the affected person is mentally or physically retarded.

infant mortality

infected *adj*
infection

infectious disease *n*
Patients with highly infectious diseases are kept on isolation wards.

inferiority complex *n*
An inferiority complex can explain unusual behaviour of one child within a group.

infertile *adj*
infertility
The woman wished to have children and went to the doctor for treatment against infertility.

inflammation *n*
Inflammation causes the affected areas to be red in colour, hence the use of the word (from "flame") to describe this condition.

influenza *n*

Infantilismus
Infantilismus ist eine psychische Behinderung, wobei die betroffene Person entweder geistig oder körperlich eingeschränkt ist.
Säuglingssterblichkeit

infiziert
Infektion

ansteckende Krankheit
Patienten mit stark übertragbaren Krankheiten werden auf einer Isolierstation untergebracht.

Minderwertigkeitskomplex
Ein Minderwertigkeitskomplex kann das ungewöhnliche Verhalten eines Kindes in der Gruppe erklären.

unfruchtbar
Unfruchtbarkeit
Die Frau wünschte sich Kinder und ging deshalb zum Arzt, um sich wegen Unfruchtbarkeit behandeln zu lassen.

Entzündung
Entzündete Bereiche sind rotfarbig, daher wird das Wort „inflammation" (von „Flamme") hier verwendet.

Grippe

Influenza is an acute viral infection, for which the incubation period lasts about three days, and the disease itself between three and ten days. It affects the respiratory tract.

infusion *n*
One example of an infusion is a saline solution.
inhale *v*
Inhaling helps, when you have a cold.
inhalant

inject *v*
injection

Infusion
Als Infusion gilt zum Beispiel eine Salzwasserlösung.
inhalieren
Inhalieren hilft bei Schnupfen.
Inhalationsmittel

einspritzen
Spritze

The nurse gave me an injection. | Die Krankenschwester gab mir eine Spritze.

inlay *n*
Inlays are very expensive.

Inlay
Inlays sind sehr teuer.

inner ear *n*
An inner ear infection can be dangerous.

Innenohr
Eine Innenohrinfektion kann gefährlich sein.

in-patient *n*
He was an in-patient of the geriatric ward.

stationärer Patient
Er war Patient auf der Station für Geriatrie.

insane *adj*
The criminal was pronounced insane.

insanity

geisteskrank
Der Kriminelle wurde für geisteskrank erklärt.
Wahnsinn, Geisteskrankheit

insomnia *n*
The insomnia was due to stress at work.

Schlaflosigkeit
Die Schlaflosigkeit war auf Stress bei der Arbeit zurückzuführen.

instinct *n*
Humans also have animal instincts.

Trieb
Auch Menschen haben tierische Triebe.

insulin *n*
For some diabetics, diet is sufficient; others have to inject insulin.

insulin shock

Insulin
Bei manchen Diabetikern genügt es, die Essgewohnheiten umzustellen, andere müssen Insulin spritzen.
Insulinschock

intensive care *n*
intensive care unit
She worked in the intensive care unit for three years.

Intensivpflege
Intensivstation
Sie arbeitete drei Jahre lang auf der Intensivstation.

internal specialist *n*
The GP advised the patient to see an internal specialist.

Internist
Der Hausarzt riet dem Patienten, einen Internisten zu konsultieren.

intestines *n*
The intestines are part of the alimentary canal.

Eingeweide
Die Eingeweide sind Teil des Verdauungskanals.

intoxication *n*
intoxicated
The blood test revealed that the car driver was intoxicated.

Intoxikation
betrunken
Der Bluttest zeigte, dass der Autofahrer betrunken war.

intravenous *adj*
The patient was given an intravenous injection.

intravenös
Der Patient bekam eine intravenöse Spritze.

involuntary *adj*
We do not have conscious control over involuntary muscle movements.

unwillkürlich, vegetativ
Wir haben keine bewusste Kontrolle über unwillkürliche Muskelbewegungen.

iodine *n*
Lack of iodine affects the thyroid gland functions.

Jod
Jodmangel beeinträchtigt die Funktionen der Schilddrüse.

iris *n*
The iris surrounds the pupil of the eye.

Iris
Die Iris umhüllt die Pupille.

iron deficiency *n*
Iron deficiency occurs, for example, in women with heavy periods.

Eisenmangel
Eisenmangel tritt zum Beispiel bei Frauen mit starken Monatsblutungen auf.

itchiness *n*
Itchiness can be associated with some skin rashes.
itch

Juckreiz
Juckreiz tritt bei manchen Hautausschlägen auf.
jucken

J/K/L

jaundice *n*
The typical yellow skin colour associated with jaundice is caused by bile pigments.

Gelbsucht
Die typisch gelbe Hautfarbe bei Gelbsucht wird durch Gallenpigmente verursacht.

jawbone *n*
The technical term for jawbone is mandible.

Kiefer
Der technische Begriff für den Hauptknochen des Kiefers ist „Mandibel".

jetlag *n*
Jetlag is a problem faced by many business people who travel around the world.

Jetlag
Der Jetlag stellt für viele Geschäftsleute, die um die Welt reisen, ein Problem dar.

joint *n*
The hip joint is a ball-and-socket joint.
joint capsule

Gelenk
Das Hüftgelenk ist ein Kugelgelenk.
Gelenkkapsel

juvenile *adj*
The juvenile court decided the boy should see a psychologist.

jugendlich
Das Jugendgericht entschied, der Junge solle zum Psychologen.

kidney *n*
The kidney donor was a man who had died in a bus crash.
kidney stone

Niere
Der Nierenspender war ein Mann, der bei einem Busunfall ums Leben kam.
Nierenstein

knee *n*
knee cap
He injured his knee cap playing football.

Knie
Kniescheibe
Er verletzte sich beim Fußballspielen die Kniescheibe.

knee joint *n*
knee ligaments

Kniegelenk
Kniebänder

knuckle *n*
He grazed his knuckles against the wall.

Knöchel
Er schürfte sich die Knöchel an der Wand ab.

label *n*
Before taking drugs, you should read the label and the instructions carefully.

Etikett
Bevor man Medikamente nimmt, sollte man das Etikett und die Anleitung sorgfältig lesen.

laboratory *n*
Specimens are sent to a laboratory for testing.

Labor
Proben werden zur Untersuchung ins Labor geschickt.

labour *n*
labour pains
When she was admitted to hospital, the labour pains were coming regularly (every few minutes).

Wehen, Geburt
Wehen
Als sie ins Krankenhaus eingeliefert wurde, kamen die Wehen regelmäßig alle paar Minuten.

laceration *n*
lacerate
His arm was badly lacerated.

Risswunde, Einriss
aufschlitzen
Er hatte schlimme Risswunden am Arm.

lacrimal gland *n*
The lacrimal glands produce tears which keep the eyes moist.

Tränendrüse
Die Tränendrüsen produzieren Tränenflüssigkeit, die die Augen feucht halten.

lactation *n*
lactating
A lactating mother should drink plenty of fluids to replace what the baby takes.

Säugen, Stillzeit
stillend
Eine stillende Mutter soll viel trinken, um die von ihrem Kind aufgenommene Flüssigkeit zu ersetzen.

lactic acid *n*
Lactic acid is the acid contained in milk.

Milchsäure
Milchsäure ist, wie der Name sagt, in Milch enthalten.

laparoscopy *n*
The patient had been suffering from severe abdominal pain, and so the doctors performed a laparoscopy.

Laparoskopie
Der Patient hatte an starken Bauchschmerzen gelitten und die Ärzte führten deswegen eine Laparoskopie durch.

laser *n*
There are many applications of laser technology in surgery.
laser therapy

Laser
Lasertechnologie wird in der Chirurgie vielfach eingesetzt.
Lasertherapie

latex *n*
Condoms are made of latex.

Latex
Kondome werden aus Latex hergestellt.

laxative *n*
The GP prescribed a mild laxative.

Abführmittel
Der Hausarzt verschrieb ein leichtes Abführmittel.

learning disorder *n*
The ten-year old was having difficulties at school due to a learning disorder.

Lernstörung
Der Zehnjährige hatte aufgrund einer Lernstörung Schwierigkeiten in der Schule.

lecithin *n*
Lecithin is used, among other things, in the production of cosmetics.

Lezithin
Lezithin wird unter anderem bei der Herstellung von Kosmetika verwendet.

legalisation *n*
The legalisation of certain drugs is a controversial topic.

Legalisierung
Die Legalisierung bestimmter Drogen ist ein kontrovers diskutiertes Thema.

lens *n*
He took his glasses to the optician to have the lenses changed.

Linse, Brillenglas
Er brachte seine Brille zum Optiker, um die Gläser auswechseln zu lassen.

leper *n*
We read about lepers in the Bible.
leprosy
leper hospital

Leprakranker
Wir lesen in der Bibel über Leprakranke.
Lepra
Leprakrankenhaus

lethal *adj*
lethal dose
The man died of a lethal dose of morphine.

tödlich
tödliche Dosis
Der Mann starb an einer tödlichen Dosis Morphium.

lethargy *n*
lethargic
She was feeling too lethargic to do anything energetic.
lethargic encephalitis

Lethargie
träge
Sie fühlte sich zu träge, um etwas zu unternehmen.
europäische Schlafkrankheit

leucocyte *n*
The leucocytes are the white blood corpuscles.

Leukozyt
Die Leukozyten sind die weißen Blutkörperchen.

leukaemia *n*
One symptom of leukaemia is an excess of leucocytes.

Leukämie, Blutkrebs
Ein Symptom von Leukämie ist ein Übermaß an Leukozyten.

libido *n*
Loss of libido may have a number of causes.

Libido
Der Verlust der Libido kann verschiedenste Ursachen haben.

lie *v*
She was lying in bed when the doctor arrived.

liegen
Sie lag im Bett, als der Arzt ankam.

life *n*
life expectancy
Life expectancy is longer for women than for men.
lifeless

Leben
Lebenserwartung
Die Lebenserwartung ist bei Frauen höher als bei Männern.
leblos

lifesaving *adj*
Thanks to the lifesaving efforts of the passers-by, the man survived the accident.

lebensrettend
Dank der lebensrettenden Maßnahmen der Passanten überlebte der Mann den Unfall.

life-threatening *n*
Cancer need not be a life-threatening disease, if diagnosed in good time.

lebensbedrohlich
Krebs muss nicht unbedingt eine lebensbedrohliche Krankheit sein, wenn sie früh erkannt wird.

ligament *n*
He tore a ligament.

Band
Er hat sich ein Band gezerrt.

ligature *n*
A ligature stops the flow of blood.

Abbinden
Das Abbinden hemmt die Blutung.

light headed *adj*
She was feeling light-headed, as she left the room.

benommen
Sie fühlte sich benommen, als sie aus dem Zimmer ging.

limb *n*
Limb is the general term for the arms and legs.

Glied
Glied ist der allgemeine Begriff für Arme und Beine.

liniment *n*
A liniment is applied externally to relieve pain.

Einreibemittel
Ein Einreibemittel wird äußerlich aufgetragen, um Schmerzen zu lindern.

linoleic acid *n*
Linoleic acid is used in the manufacture of soap.

lip *n*
His lips were very dry.

lipid *n*
Lipids form particles called liposomes.

liposome

lip-read *v*
Deaf people are able to lip-read.

liquid *n*
A liquid diet was recommended.

lisp *v*
I used to lisp slightly as a child, but now I have managed to cure this.

listless *n*
She was so listless, I assumed she was depressed.
listlessness

litmus *n*
Litmus paper is used in chemistry.

liver n

Linolsäure
Linolsäure wird bei der Herstellung von Seife verwendet.

Lippe
Seine Lippen waren sehr trocken.

Lipid
Lipide bilden Partikel, die Liposome heißen.
Liposom

ablesen, von den Lippen lesen
Taube können von den Lippen ablesen.

Flüssigkeit
Flüssigkost wurde empfohlen.

lispeln
Ich habe als Kind ein wenig gelispelt, aber jetzt ist es mir gelungen, dies einzustellen.

teilnahmslos
Sie war so teilnahmslos, dass ich sie für depressiv hielt.
Teilnahmslosigkeit

Lackmus
Lackmuspapier wird in der Chemie verwendet.

Leber

The **liver** has many functions, including the storage of glycogen and the detoxification of poisons. It also secretes bile and maintains a constant level of nutrients in the body.

local *adj*
The dentist gave his patient a local anaesthetic.

logopaedics *n*
Logopaedics is speech therapy.

longevity *n*
It is questionable whether longevity is desirable or not.

örtlich
Der Zahnarzt gab dem Patienten eine örtliche Betäubung.

Logopädie
Logopädie ist Sprachtherapie.

Langlebigkeit
Es ist fraglich, ob es wünschenswert ist, lange zu leben oder nicht.

long-term *adj*
long-term treatment
Long-term treatment is necessary for some incurable diseases.

Dauer-
Dauerbehandlung
Eine Dauerbehandlung ist bei manchen unheilbaren Krankheiten erforderlich.

louse *n*
The children were sent home from the kindergarten because they had lice in their hair.

Laus
Die Kinder wurden vom Kindergarten nach Hause geschickt, weil sie Läuse im Haar hatten.

low calorie *adj*
There are plenty of low calorie drinks available for people on a diet.

kalorienarm
Es gibt viele kalorienarme Getränke für Leute, die abnehmen wollen.

low-fat *adj*
Low-fat milk is recommended.

fettarm
Fettarme Milch wird empfohlen.

lubricant *n*
The gynaecologist can prescribe a lubricant.

Gleitmittel
Der Frauenarzt kann ein Gleitmittel verschreiben.

lumbago *n*
The pain in the lower back associated with lumbago makes it difficult for sufferers to walk.

Hexenschuss
Ein durch Hexenschuss ausgelöster Schmerz in der Lendengegend erschwert das Gehen.

lumbar puncture *n*
A lumbar puncture is performed to withdraw fluid or to administer drugs.

Lumbalpunktion
Eine Lumbalpunktion wird durchgeführt, um Körperflüssigkeit zu entnehmen oder Medikamente einzuspritzen.

lymph node *n*
The function of the lymph nodes is to protect us against infection.

Lymphknoten
Es ist die Funktion der Lymphknoten, uns gegen Infektionen zu schützen.

lymphatic system *n*
lymphatic vessels

lymphatisches System
Lymphgefäße

macrobiotic *adj*
A macrobiotic diet excludes all animal products.

makrobiotisch
Eine makrobiotische Diät schließt alle Tierprodukte aus.

mad cow disease *n*
Mad cow disease is another term for BSE.

Rinderwahn
Rinderwahn ist ein anderer Begriff für BSE.

malformation *n*
Malformation of a part of the body is usually congenital.

Fehlbildung
Die Fehlbildung eines Körperteils ist üblicherweise ein Geburtsfehler.

malignant *adj*
Thank goodness the tumour was not malignant!

bösartig
Der Tumor war Gott sei Dank nicht bösartig!

malnutrition *n*
Many inhabitants of the third world are suffering from malnutrition.

Mangelernährung
Viele Einheimische der Dritten Welt leiden unter Mangelernährung.

malpractice *n*
The doctor was accused of malpractice.

Kunstfehler
Dem Arzt wurde ein Kunstfehler vorgeworfen.

maltreatment *n*

Misshandlung

mammary gland *n*
The mammary glands are stimulated by the baby sucking to produce milk.

Milchdrüse
Durch das Saugen des Babys werden die Milchdrüsen zur Milchproduktion angeregt.

mammography *n*
The gynaecologist recommended a mammography, since the patient was taking hormones.

Mammographie
Der Frauenarzt empfahl eine Mammographie, da die Patientin Hormone nahm.

mandible *n*
Mandible is the technical term for jawbone.

Kiefer
„Mandibel" ist der technische Begriff für Kiefer.

mania *n*
Mania is a mental disorder which can lead to violence.
mania of persecution

Manie
Manie ist eine psychische Krankheit, die manchmal zu Gewalt führen kann.
Verfolgungswahn

manic-depressive *adj*
Manic-depressive patients are either euphoric or deeply depressive.

manisch-depressiv
Manisch depressive Patienten sind entweder euphorisch oder tief deprimiert.

manipulate *v*
A chiropractor manipulates the spine to relieve pain.

manipulieren
Ein Chiropraktiker manipuliert die Wirbelsäule, um Schmerzen zu lindern.

marrow *n*
bone marrow
marrow activity

Mark
Knochenmark
Markaktivität

masculine *adj*
Some characteristics are particularly masculine.

maskulin
Einige Eigenschaften sind besonders maskulin.

masochism *n*
masochist
Masochists derive pleasure from inflicting suffering on themselves.

Masochismus
Masochist
Masochisten empfinden Freude, indem sie sich selbst bestrafen.

massage *m*
Many beauty salons offer facial or body massage.
masseur

Massage
Viele Kosmetiksalons bieten Gesichts- oder Körpermassage an.
Masseur

mastectomy *n*
The patient was relieved to hear she did not need to undergo a mastectomy.

Brustamputation
Die Patientin war erleichtert zu hören, dass sie sich keiner Brustamputation unterziehen müsse.

mastication *n*
Mastication is good exercise for gums and teeth.
masticate

Kauen
Kauen ist ein gutes Trainig für Zahnfleisch und Zähne.
kauen

masturbation *n*
masturbate
My boyfriend masturbated regularly.

Onanie
masturbieren
Mein Freund masturbierte regelmäßig.

maternity ward *n*
There were fifty mothers in the maternity ward.
maternity leave

Entbindungsstation
Es waren fünfzig Mütter auf der Entbindungsstation.
Kinderpause, Erziehungsurlaub

mature *adj*
She was very mature for her age.

reif
Sie war für ihr Alter sehr reif.

meal *n*
Hospital meals are not very appetizing.

Mahlzeit
Die Mahlzeiten im Krankenhaus sind nicht sehr appetitanregend.

medical *adj*
I decided to take out private medical insurance.
medical attendance
medical card

medizinisch
Ich entschloss mich, eine private Krankenversicherung abzuschließen.
ärztliche Behandlung
Krankenunterlagen

medical certificate *n*
He needed a medical certificate for his employer.

Attest
Er benötigte ein Attest für seinen Arbeitgeber.

medical profession *n*

A nurse is a member of the medical profession.

Oberbegriff für die medizinischen Berufe
Krankenschwester ist ein medizinischer Beruf.

---

medical record *n*
I once worked in the medical records department of one of the London hospitals.
Medical Register

Krankenbericht
Ich war einmal in der Krankenbericht-Abteilung eines der Londoner Krankenhäuser beschäftigt.
Ärzteregister

---

medical science *n*

Medical science will surely progress dramatically over the next ten years.

die medizinischen Wissenschaften, Heilkunde
Die Medizin wird sicherlich im Laufe der nächsten zehn Jahre riesen Fortschritte erzielen.

---

medical student *n*
Medical students have to accustom themselves to the sight of blood.

Medizinstudent
Medizinstudenten müssen sich daran gewöhnen, Blut zu sehen.

---

medication *n*
Don't forget to take your medication!

Medikament, Arznei
Vergiss nicht, deine Medikamente zu nehmen!

---

medicinal *adj*
Medicinal herbs can be an alternative to conventional medicines.

medizinisch, Heil-
Heilkräuter können eine Alternative zur herkömmlichen Medizin darstellen.

---

medicine *n*
On the medicine bottle it said, "Take two teaspoons after meals".

Medizin
Auf der Medizinflasche stand: „Nehmen Sie zwei Teelöffel nach den Mahlzeiten".

---

megalomania *n*
Symptomatic of megalomania is the illusion of power and wealth.

Größenwahn
Symptomatisch für Größenwahn ist die Illusion von Macht und Reichtum.

---

melanoma *n*
A melanoma is a malignant skin tumour.

Melanom
Ein Melanom ist ein bösartiger Hauttumor.

---

membrane *n*
The lining of an organ is called a membrane.

Membran
Die Innenschicht eines Organs wird als Membran bezeichnet.

---

memory *n*
They say one's memory deteriorates as one gets older.
memory loss

Gedächtnis
Angeblich verschlechtert sich das Gedächtnis mit dem Alter.
Gedächtnisverlust

Mendel's laws *n, pl*
Mendel's laws are the laws which govern heredity.

Mendel-Gesetz
Das Mendel-Gesetz beschreibt die Vererbung.

meningitis *n*
Meningitis is a serious illness resulting from infection.

Gehirnhautentzündung
Eine Gehirnhautentzündung ist eine ernsthafte, durch Infektion verursachte Krankheit.

meniscus *n*
He injured his meniscus.
meniscus cyst

Meniskus
Er verletzte sich am Meniskus.
Meniskuszyste

menopause *n*

Wechseljahre

The typical symptoms of the **menopause,** hot flushes, depression, difficulty sleeping and osteoporosis, can be alleviated by HRT, i. e. Hormone Replacement Therapy.

menorrhalgia *n*
Many women suffer from the cramp-like pains of menorrhalgia.

Periodenschmerz
Viele Frauen leiden unter krampfhaften Periodenschmerzen.

menstrual cycle *n*
The menstrual cycle lasts approximately twenty-eight days.

Menstruationszyklus
Der Menstruationszyklus beträgt ungefähr achtundzwanzig Tage.

menstruation *n*
Menstruation begins during puberty between about eleven and thirteen years of age.

Menstruation
Die Menstruation beginnt während der Pubertät zwischen etwa elf und dreizehn Jahren.

mental *adj*
The rapist was suffering from a serious mental disorder.

psychisch
Der Vergewaltiger war schwer geistesgestört.

mentally handicapped *adj*
We visited a school for the mentally handicapped.

geistig behindert
Wir besuchten eine Schule für geistig Behinderte.

menthol *n*
Menthol is a good remedy for colds.

Menthol
Menthol ist ein gutes Heilmittel bei Erkältung.

metabolic rate *n*
The metabolic rate denotes the speed of all the chemical processes carried out by the body.

Stoffwechselumsatz
Der Stoffwechselumsatz verzeichnet die Geschwindigkeit aller chemischen Prozesse des Körpers.

metastasis *n*
When cancer spreads from one part of the body to others, this process is referred to as "metastasis".

Metastasen
Wenn sich Krebs auf andere Körperteile ausbreitet, nennt man diesen Prozess „Metastasenbildung".

microbe *n*
A microbe is a microscopic organism which can spread disease.

Mikrobe
Eine Mikrobe ist ein mikroskopischer Organismus, der Krankheiten verbreiten kann.

microscope *n*
He examined the specimen under the microscope.

Mikroskop
Er untersuchte die Probe unter dem Mikroskop.

midwife *n*
The local midwife delivered my second baby.

Hebamme
Die Hebamme unseres Stadtteils brachte mein zweites Kind zur Welt.

migraine *n*
Food allergies can be responsible for migraine attacks.

Migräne
Lebensmittelallergien können für Migräneanfälle verantwortlich sein.

milk *n*
Allowing the baby to suck, and drinking plenty, should ensure the milk flow.

Milch
Das Saugen des Babys sowie ausreichende Flüssigkeitszufuhr sorgt für den Milchfluss der Mutter.

milk tooth *n*
Babies are often irritable when they are cutting their milk teeth.

Milchzahn
Babys sind oft quengelig, wenn sie ihre Milchzähne bekommen.

miracle drug *n*
Babyboomers are hoping for the miracle drug which will stop them ageing.

Wundermittel
Babyboomer hoffen auf ein Wundermittel, das ihren Alterungsprozess stoppen wird.

miscarriage *n*
Her first pregnancy ended in a miscarriage, but then she gave birth to a beautiful baby girl.

Fehlgeburt
Ihre erste Schwangerschaft endete in einer Fehlgeburt, aber dann bekam sie ein wunderschönes Mädchen.

morning sickness *n*
A cup of tea and a biscuit before getting up, helps prevent morning sickness.

Schwangerschaftserbrechen
Eine Tasse Tee mit Keks vor dem Aufstehen hilft gegen Schwangerschaftserbrechen am Morgen.

morphine *n*
His father was given morphine in the latter stages of cancer.

Morphium
Sein Vater bekam Morphium in den letzten Stadien von Krebs.

mortality rate *n*
*The mortality rate for heart attacks is
high in industrialized countries.*

Sterberate
*Die Sterberate für Herzinfarkte ist in den
Industrieländern hoch.*

mother's milk *n*
*If a mother wants to leave her baby with
a babysitter, she can express milk be-
forehand, so the baby still gets mother's
milk and not formula.*

Muttermilch
*Wenn eine Mutter einen Babysitter
engagieren möchte, kann sie Milch
abpumpen, damit ihr Baby dennoch
Muttermilch und keine Fertignahrung
bekommt.*

mouth-to-mouth resuscitation *n*
*The policeman gave mouth-to-mouth
resuscitation until the ambulance arrived,
which saved the man's life.*

Mund-zu-Mund-Beatmung
*Der Polizist vollzog eine lebensrettende
Mund-zu-Mund Beatmung, bis der Kran-
kenwagen ankam.*

mucous *adj*
*Membranes lining various organs secrete
mucous.*
mucous gland
mucous plug

schleimabsondernd
*Die innere Schicht sämtlicher Organe
besteht aus Schleimhaut.*
Schleimdrüse
Schleimpfropf

mucous membranes *n*
mucus

Schleimhaut
Schleim

multiple birth *n*
*Fertility drugs have resulted in multiple
births.*

Mehrfachgeburt
*Fruchtbarkeitsmedikamente haben
Mehrfachgeburten herbeigeführt.*

multiple sclerosis *n*
*Multiple sclerosis affects the central
nervous system.*

Multiple-Sklerose
*Multiple-Sklerose betrifft das zentrale
Nervensystem.*

mumps *n*
Mumps is a childhood disease.

Mumps
Mumps ist eine Kinderkrankheit.

muscle *n*
He pulled a muscle in his arm.
muscle belly
muscle cramp
muscle fibre
to strain a muscle

Muskel
Er zerrte sich einen Muskel im Arm.
Muskelbauch
Muskelkrampf
Muskelfaser
einen Muskel zerren

mutism *n*
Mutism is the inability to speak.

Stummheit
*Stummheit ist die Unfähigkeit zu
sprechen.*

myopia *n*
Myopia is short-sightedness.

Myopie
Myopie ist Kurzsichtigkeit.

nail *n*
She had an ingrowing toenail.

Nagel
Sie hatte einen eingewachsenen Zehennagel.

---

naked *adj*
Since her husband went out into the street naked, she finally had to admit that he needed psychiatric help.

nackt
Erst als ihr Mann nackt auf die Straße ging, musste sie zugeben, dass er psychatrische Hilfe brauchte.

---

nappy *n*
The young mothers were shown how to change their babies' nappies.

Windel
Man zeigte den jungen Müttern, wie man ein Baby wickelt.

---

narcissism *n*
Narcissism is a preoccupation with one's own appearance.

Narzissmus
Narzissmus ist die ständige Beschäftigung mit dem eigenen Aussehen.

---

narcosis *n*
narcosis therapy
narcostimulant

Narkose
Schlaftherapie
Narkostimulans

---

narcotic *n*
Narcotics are powerful drugs which relieve pain, but are also used by drug addicts.

Narkotikum, Rauschgift
Narkotika sind starke Drogen, die Schmerzen lindern, die aber auch von Drogenabhängigen genommen werden.

---

narrowing *n*
Narrowing of the arteries occurs as people get older.

Verengung
Eine Verengung der Arterien findet im höheren Alter statt.

---

nasal *n*
nasal cavity
When one has a head cold, the nasal cavities are blocked with mucus.
nasoscopy

nasal
Nasenhöhle
Beim Schnupfen sind die Nasenhöhlen mit Schleim verstopft.
Nasenspiegelung

---

natural *adj*
The women were in favour of natural childbirth.

natürlich
Die Frauen hatten sich für den natürlichen Geburtsvorgang entschieden.

---

naturopathy *n*
Naturopathy embraces many different areas and methods, such as kinesiology or the use of oils and Bach flowers.

Naturheilkunde
Die Naturheilkunde schließt viele Bereiche und Methoden ein, z. B. Kinesiologie oder den Einsatz von Ölen und Bachblüten.

nausea *n*
She complained of nausea and loss of appetite.

Übelkeit
Sie klagte über Übelkeit und Appetitlosigkeit.

navel *n*
My daughter has a pierced navel.

Nabel
Meine Tochter hat einen Bauchnabelpiercing.

neck *n*
She had a stiff neck from sitting in a draught all evening.

Nacken
Ihr Nacken war steif, weil sie den ganzen Abend im Luftzug gesessen hatte.

needle *n*
Needle is an abbreviation of hypodermic needle, meaning a syringe.

Nadel
Im medizinischen Sinn bezieht sich das Wort „Nadel" auf eine Spritze.

negligence *n*
The hospital was sued for negligence, but was subsequently acquitted.

Nachlässigkeit
Das Krankenhaus wurde wegen Nachlässigkeit verklagt, aber anschließend freigesprochen.

nerve *n*
The nerves transmit impulses to the brain and spinal cord.

Nerv
Die Nerven übermitteln Impulse an Gehirn und Wirbelsäule.

nervous breakdown *n*
She had a nervous breakdown two years ago, and has been attending therapy since then.

Nervenzusammenbruch
Sie hatte vor zwei Jahren einen Nervenzusammenbruch und ist seitdem in Therapie.

nervous system *n*
The nervous system is the body's sensory mechanism.

Nervensystem
Das Nervensystem ist der Sensormechanismus des Körpers.

nettle rash *n*
Nettle rash is the popular term for urticaria.

Nesselsucht
„Urticaria" wird in der Laiensprache als „Nesselsucht" bezeichnet.

neuralgia *n*
When a nerve is injured, the resulting pain is referred to as neuralgia.

Neuralgie
Wenn man einen Nerv verletzt, nennt man die damit verbundenen Schmerzen „Neuralgie".

neurodermatitis *n*
Neurodermatitis produces an itchy skin rash.

Neurodermitis
Neurodermitis erzeugt einen Hautausschlag mit Juckreiz.

neurology *n*
neurologist

Neurologie
Neurologe

neurosis *n*
neurotic
We call someone neurotic, when their unusual behaviour, and possible over-anxiety, has no logical reason.

neurotic

Neurose
neurotisch
Wir nennen eine Person neurotisch, deren ungewöhnliches Benehmen und exzessive Nervosität keine logische Begründung hat.
Neurotiker

newborn *adj*
We usually place newborn babies on their side, since they cannot yet turn over themselves.
newborn care
newborn jaundice
newborn mortality rate
newborn nursery

neugeboren
Wir legen neugeborene Babys seitlich ins Bett, da sie sich noch nicht von alleine umdrehen können.
Neugeborenenpflege
Neugeborenengelbsucht
Neugeborenensterblichkeitsrate
Neugeborenenpflege

night-blind *adj*
She had difficulty driving at night, because she was night-blind.

nachtblind
Sie hatte Schwierigkeiten beim Auto-fahren in der Nacht, da sie nachtblind war.

nickel allergy *n*
Costume jewellery is usually nickel-free these days, because a nickel allergy is very common.

Nickelallergie
Modeschmuck ist heutzutage meistens nickelfrei, weil Nickelallergie sehr häufig vorkommt.

nicotine *n*
Nicotine tablets are issued to smokers during non-smoking, transatlantic flights.

Nikotin
Rauchern werden während Nicht-raucherflügen Nikotintabletten angeboten.

night duty *n*
My friend is a nurse and she is on night duty next week.

Nachtdienst
Meine Freundin ist Krankenschwes-ter und hat nächste Woche Nacht-dienst.

night nurse *n*
The patient had difficulty sleeping, and called for the night nurse to give him a sleeping tablet.

Nachtschwester
Der Patient litt an Schlafstörungen und rief die Nachtschwester, um eine Schlaf-tablette zu bekommen.

nipple *n*
Breastfeeding mothers should take care of their nipples.

Brustwarze
Stillende Mütter sollten ihre Brustwarzen pflegen.

non-toxic *adj*
It is possible to buy non-toxic household cleansing products.

ungiftig
Man kann ungiftiges Putzmittel kaufen.

nose drops *n, pl*
Nose drops help when you have a cold.

nose *n*
nosebleed
The child often had severe nosebleeds.
nostril

nurse *n*
She was a nurse in one of the big London teaching hospitals.

nursing home *n*
The patient was transferred to a nursing home to convalesce.

nursing period *n*
The Americans refer to breastfeeding as "nursing"; the nursing period is therefore the period during which a baby is breastfed.

nutrient *n*
One should ensure that one's diet contains all the essential nutrients.

nutrition *n*
Good nutrition is essential for a healthy body.
nutritive value

nymphomania *n*
nymphomaniac
Nymphomaniacs do not have lasting relationships.

obese *n*
The obese woman weighed almost eighty kilogrammes.
obesity

observation *n*
The patient was taken into hospital for observation.

Nasentropfen
Nasentropfen helfen beim Schnupfen.

Nase
Nasenbluten
Das Kind hatte oft starkes Nasenbluten.
Nasenloch

Krankenschwester
Sie war Krankenschwester in einem der großen Londoner Ausbildungskranken-häuser.

Pflegeheim
Der Patient wurde in ein Pflegeheim überwiesen, um sich zu erholen.

Stillzeit
Die Amerikaner nennen den Vorgang des Stillens „nursing". „nursing period" ist daher der Zeitraum, während dessen ein Baby gestillt wird.

Nährstoff
Man sollte sicherstellen, dass die Diät alle erforderlichen Nährstoffe enthält.

Ernährung
Eine gute Ernährung ist für einen gesunden Körper unentbehrlich.
Nährwert

Nymphomanie
Nymphomanin
Nymphomaninnen führen keine länge-ren, partnerschaftlichen Beziehungen.

fettleibig
Die fettleibige Frau wog fast achzig Kilogramm.
Fettleibigkeit

Überwachung, Kontrolle
Der Patient wurde zur Kontrolle ins Krankenhaus eingeliefert.

obstetrician *n*
obstetrics
Obstetrics is the branch of medicine concerned with childbirth.

Geburtshelfer
Obstetrik, Geburtshilfe
Obstetrik ist der medizinische Bereich, der sich mit der Geburt befasst.

occlusion *n*
We produce occlusion when we chew, or close the vocal tract in order to utter a plosiv.

Verschluss
Wir verschließen den Kiefer als Teil des Kauvorgangs oder den Vokaltrakt, um einen Verschlusslaut zu artikulieren.

occupational therapy *n*
Occupational therapy helps patients to regain the use of weakened muscles.

Beschäftigungstherapie
Beschäftigungstherapie hilft Patienten, geschwächte Muskeln wieder sicher zu benutzen.

odontology *n*
Odontology is the branch of medicine concerned with teeth.

Zahnmedizin, Odontologie, Zahnheilkunde
Odontologie ist der medizinische Bereich, der sich mit den Zähnen befasst.

oedema *n*
Oedema is the condition whereby fluid accumulates between tissue cells.

Ödem
Ein Ödem ist der Zustand, worin sich Flüssigkeit zwischen den Gewebezellen sammelt.

oesophagus *n*
Food passes to the stomach through the oesophagus.

Speiseröhre
Nahrung wird durch die Speiseröhre zum Magen transportiert.

oestrogen *n*
The production of oestrogen decreases with age.

Östrogen
Die Östrogenproduktion verringert sich mit dem Alter.

of unsound mind *adj*
The witness was pronounced of unsound mind, after numerous psychological tests.

unzurechnungsfähig
Nach zahlreichen psychologischen Tests wurde der Zeuge für unzurechnungsfähig erklärt.

ointment *n*
The skin specialist prescribed some ointment.

Salbe
Der Hautarzt verschrieb eine Salbe.

olfactory nerve *n*
The olfactory nerve is connected to the mucous membranes of the nose.

Riechnerv
Der Riechnerv ist mit der Nasenschleimhaut verbunden.

on-call *adj*
The doctor was on-call last weekend.

auf Abruf
Der Arzt hatte letztes Wochenende Bereitschaftsdienst.

oncology *n*
oncologist
An oncologist is a cancer specialist.

Onkologie
Onkologe
Ein Onkologe ist ein Krebsspezialist.

open-heart surgery *n*
In order to perform open-heart surgery, the blood circulation is maintained by machinery.

offene Herzchirurgie
Um offene Herzchirurgie durchzuführen, wird die Blutzirkulation durch Maschinen erhalten.

operation *n*
She went into hospital last week to have an operation on her knee.
operating theatre

Operation
Sie ging letzte Woche ins Krankenhaus, um ihr Knie operieren zu lassen.
Operationssaal

opthalmia *n*
Inflammation of the eyes is called opthalmia.

Augenentzündung
Der lateinische Begriff „opthalmia" bezieht sich auf eine Augenentzündung.

optic nerve *n*
The optic nerve connects the retina to the brain.

Sehnerv
Der Sehnerv verbindet die Netzhaut mit dem Gehirn.

optician *n*
He went to the optician, because he needed reading glasses.

Augenoptiker
Er ging zum Augenoptiker, weil er eine Lesebrille benötigte.

Oral vaccination *n*
Oral vaccination is common against polio.

Schluckimpfung
Eine Schluckimpfung gegen Polio ist üblich.

organ *n*
The blood carries oxygen and nutrients to the major organs, and to other parts of the body.
organ donation

Organ
Das Blut liefert Sauer- und Nährstoff zu den Hauptorganen und anderen Körperteilen.
Organspende

orthodontist *n*
Orthodontist is another term for dental orthopaedist.

Kieferorthopäde
Die englische Sprache hat zwei Begriffe für den Kieferorthopäden: „orthodontist" und „dental orthopaedist".

orthopaedics *n*
orthopaedist
Patients with spinal problems or problems with their joints visit the orthopaedist.

Orthopädie
Orthopäde
Patienten mit Problemen an der Wirbelsäule oder in den Gelenken besuchen den Orthopäden.

osteoarthritis *n*

Osteoarthritis, Gelenkentzündung

Osteoarthritis is a degenerative disease of the joints causing pain and stiffness, usually in elderly people. The symptoms are worsened by prolonged activity.

osteoporosis *n*
Osteoporosis is characterised by a reduction in bone mass, causing bones to fracture more easily.

Osteoporose
Osteoporose wird durch eine Reduktion der Knochenmasse charakerisiert, was dazu führt, dass die Knochen leichter brechen.

outpatients' department *n*
National Health patients are often faced with long waiting times in outpatients' departments.

Ambulanz
Gesetzlich Versicherte werden in England oft mit langen Wartezeiten in der Ambulanz konfrontiert.

ovary *n*
Oestrogen is secreted by the ovaries.

Eierstock
Die Eierstöcke sondern Östrogen ab.

over-active thyroid gland *n*
Two symptoms of an over-active thyroid gland are high blood pressure and increased metabolism.

Überfunktion der Schilddrüse
Zwei Symptome einer Überfunktion der Schilddrüse sind hoher Blutdruck und gesteigerter Metabolismus.

overdose *n*
My friend's flat-mate died of an overdose of heroin.

Überdosis
Der Mitbewohner eines Freundes starb an einer Überdosis Heroin.

over-the-counter *n*
Over-the-counter medicines include such products as aspirin and paracetamol.

rezeptfrei
Rezeptfreie Arzneimittel schließen Produkte wie Aspirin und Paracetamol ein.

P

pacemaker n
An artificial pacemaker controls the heartbeat when this function is no longer carried out naturally due to heart disease.

Herzschrittmacher
Ein künstlicher Herzschrittmacher bestimmt den Herzschlag, wenn diese Funktion aufgrund von Herzkrankheit nicht mehr natürlich ausgeführt wird.

paediatrics *n*
paediatric clinic
I took my daughter to the paediatric clinic for tests, when she vomited constantly as an infant.

Kinderheilkunde
Kinderklinik
Ich brachte meine Tochter zur Untersuchung in die Kinderklinik, als sie als Säugling ständig erbrach.

paeditrician
He was a paeditrician at the Royal Children's Hospital.

Kinderarzt
Er war Kinderarzt am Royal Children's Hospital.

paediatrics *n*
paediatric clinic
I took my daughter to the paediatric clinic for tests, as she vomited constantly as an infant.
paeditrician

Kinderheilkunde
Kinderklinik
Ich brachte meine Tochter in die Kinderklinik zur Untersuchung, da sie als Säugling ständig erbrach.
Kinderarzt

pain *n*
pain centre
painkiller
One should not take painkillers for more than a few days without seeking medical help
painless
The operation was painless.
painrelief
pain threshold
She had a very low pain threshold.

Schmerz
Schmerzzentrum
Schmerzmittel
Man soll Schmerzmittel nicht länger als ein paar Tage nehmen, ohne einen Arzt aufzusuchen.
schmerzlos
Die Operation war schmerzlos.
Schmerzlinderung
Schmerzgrenze
Bei ihr war die Schmerzgrenze sehr niedrig.

painful *adj*
to be painful
painful breathing

schmerzhaft
schmerzhaft sein
Schmerzen beim Atmen

palate *n*
"Palate" is the technical term for the roof of the mouth.

Gaumen
In Englisch wird der Gaumen als „Munddach" bezeichnet.

palliative *n*
A palliative relieves the symptoms of an illness, but is not a cure.

Palliativ
Ein Palliativ lindert Schmerzen, ist aber kein Heilmittel.

palpable *adj*
A tumour is palpable when it can be located by touch.
palpate

palpabel
Ein Tumor ist „palpabel", wenn er durch Tasten lokalisiert werden kann.
tasten

palpitation *n*
Palpitations are the feeling that one's heart is beating too fast or too irregularly.

Palpitation
Bei Palpitationen hat man das Gefühl, dass das Herz zu schnell oder unregelmäßig schlägt.

pancreas *n*
Insulin is produced in the pancreas.

Bauchspeicheldrüse
Insulin wird in der Bauchspeicheldrüse erzeugt.

panic *n*
She suffered from panic attacks when she was outside.

Panik
Sie litt unter Panikzuständen, wenn sie draußen war.

pap smear *n*
Gynaecologists do a pap smear test at regular intervals.

Pap-Abstrich
Frauenärzte machen in regelmäßigen Zeitabständen einen Pap-Abstrich.

paralysis *n*
paralysed
His right side was paralysed after a stroke.

Lähmung
gelähmt
Seine rechte Körperhälfte war nach einem Hirnschlag gelähmt.

paranoia *n*
Symptoms of paranoia are suspicion and mistrust or the feeling of being persecuted.
paranoiac

Paranoia
Symptome von Paranoia sind Verdächtigung, Mangel an Vertrauen oder das Gefühl, verfolgt zu werden.
Paranoiker

paraplegia *n*
paraplegic
One pupil in my class is a paraplegic.

Querschnittslähmung
Querschnittsgelähmter
Eine Schülerin in meiner Klasse ist querschnittsgelähmt.

Parkinson's disease *n*

Parkinson-Krankheit

A chronic, progressive disorder of the central nervous system, **Parkinson's disease** is characterised by tremor. Patients also experience lack of muscular coordination.

parturition *n*
Parturition is a technical term for giving birth.

Geburt
„Parturition" ist ein technischer Begriff für die Entbindung.

pastille *n*
She was sucking a pastille for her sore throat.

Lutschtablette
Sie lutschte eine Tablette gegen Halsweh.

patent medicine *n*
There is a good selection of patent medicines for coughs and colds.

Markenpräparat
Es gibt eine gute Auswahl an Markenpräparaten gegen Erkältungen und Husten.

paternity test *n*
The court ordered a paternity test to determine who was the father of the child.

Vaterschaftstest
Nach Anweisung des Gerichts musste ein Vaterschaftstest durchgeführt werden, um festzustellen, wer der Vater des Kindes war.

patient *n*
The hospital admitted ten new patients yesterday evening.
to attend a patient

pathologic *adj*
pathologic fracture
pathologic heart condition
pathologic labour activity
pathologic mendacity
pathologic mitosis
pathologic sensation

pedicure *n*
She made an appointment with the chiropodist for a pedicure.

pelvic floor *n*
Pelvic floor exercises strengthen the muscles before and after childbirth.
pelvic abscess
pelvic arrest
pelvic axis
pelvic cavity
pelvis

penis *n*
The penis is the male reproductive organ.

pericardiac *adj*
pericarditis
Pericarditis is the inflammation of the pericardium.

perineotomy *n*
A perineotomy is performed to prevent tearing as the baby's head emerges.

period *n*

periodontosis *n*
Regular teeth cleaning and visits to the dental hygienist help prevent periodontosis.

peristalsis *n*
Peristalsis enables the passage of food down the oesophagus.

Patient
Zehn neue Patienten wurden gestern abend ins Krankenhaus eingeliefert.
einen Patienten pflegen

pathologisch
pathologische Fraktur
Herzleiden
pathologische Wehentätigkeit
krankhaftes Lügen
krankhafte Zellteilung
pathologische Wahrnehmung

Fußpflege
Sie machte einen Termin beim Fußpfleger.

Beckenboden
Beckenbodengymnastik verstärkt die Muskeln vor und nach der Geburt.
Becken
Beckenabszess
Beckeneinklemmung
Beckenachse
Beckenhöhle

Penis
Der Penis ist das Fortpflanzungsorgan des Mannes.

pericardial
Pericarditis
Pericarditis ist die Entzündung des Pericardiums.

Dammschnitt
Ein Dammschnitt verhindert Risswunden bei der Geburt.

Periode

Paradontose
Regelmäßiges Zähneputzen und professionelle Reinigung helfen, Paradontose vorzubeugen.

Peristaltik
Peristaltik ermöglicht die Fortbewegung von Nahrung im Körper.

peritonitis *n*
The inner lining of the abdomen is the peritoneum; if this becomes inflamed, the condition is referred to as peritonitis.

Bauchfellentzündung
Die innere Schicht des Abdomens heißt Bauchfell; wenn das Bauchfell entzündet ist, nennt man diese Krankheit Peritonitis.

pessary *n*
One form of pessary is the contraceptive diaphragm.

Pessar
Eine Art von Pessar ist ein Diaphragma zum Schutz vor Schwangerschaft.

pharmaceutical industry *n*
The pharmaceutical industry is engaged in research as well as marketing and sales.
pharmacology

pharmazeutische Industrie
Die pharmazeutische Industrie ist sowohl in der Forschung als auch in Marketing und Verkauf tätig.
Arzneimittelkunde

pharmacy *n*
"Pharmacy" is another word for "chemist". "Chemist" is more common in British English.

Apotheke
Es gibt auf Englisch zwei Wörter für Apotheke: „Pharmacy" oder „Chemist". „Chemist" wird im britischen Englisch mehr gebraucht.

pharynx *n*
pharyngitis
Pharyngitis is inflammation of the part of the alimentary canal between the mouth and the oesophagus.

Schlund
Pharyngitis
Pharyngitis ist die Entzündung des Teils im Verdauungstrakt, der zwischen Mund und Speiseröhre liegt.

phototherapy *n*
Phototherapy is important in countries where the daylight hours are very short in winter.

Lichttherapie
Lichttherapie ist wichtig in Ländern mit sehr kurzen Tagen im Winter.

physical disability *n*
Life can be complicated for people with physical disabilities and they can often be admired for their courage.

Körperbehinderung
Das Leben kann für Leute mit körperlichen Behinderungen kompliziert sein und man kann sie oft wegen ihren Mutes bewundern.

physical therapy *n*
He had to attend physical therapy after the plaster was removed from his arm, to help regain its use.

Krankengymnastik
Er musste zur Krankengymnastik, nachdem man den Gips von seinem Arm entfernte, damit er ihn wieder benutzen konnte.

physician *n*
"Physician" is another term for a doctor.

physician on call

Arzt
Arzt heißt auf Englisch „doctor" oder auch „physician".
diensthabender Arzt

pigment *n*
Albinos have no pigment in their skin.

pigmented moles

pill *n*
Remember to take your pills before you
go to bed.
to be on the pill
pill-rolling tremor

pillow *n*
He asked the nurse for an extra pillow.

pimple *n*
Pimples are one of the unfortunate
symptoms of puberty and can cause
teenagers embarrassment.

placebo *n*
He felt much better after taking the
tablets, but maybe it was just the placebo
effect.

placenta *n*
The placenta supplies the foetus with
oxygen and nutrients.

plaque *n*
Dental hygienists remove the plaque
from the teeth.

plasma *n*
The corpuscles are suspended in the
blood plasma.

plaster *n*
His leg was in plaster.
She put a plaster on the cut.

plaster bandage
plaster boot
plaster dressing

plastic *adj*

plasticity *n*

Pigment
Albinos haben keine Pigmente in der
Haut.
Pigmentflecken

Pille
Vergiss nicht, deine Pillen zu nehmen,
bevor du ins Bett gehst.
die Pille nehmen
Pillendrehen

Kissen
Er bat die Krankenschwester um ein
zusätzliches Kissen.

Pickel
Pickel sind ein Symptom der Pubertät und
sind den Jugendlichen oft peinlich.

Plazebo
Er fühlte sich viel besser, nachdem er
die Tabletten genommen hatte, aber
vielleicht war es nur der Plazebo-
Effekt.

Plazenta
Die Plazenta liefert dem Foetus
Sauerstoff und Nahrung.

Zahnstein
Bei der professionellen Zahnreinigung
wird Zahnstein entfernt.

Plasma
Die Blutkörperchen sind im Blutplasma
suspendiert.

Gips, Pflaster
Er hatte ein Gipsbein.
Sie klebte ein Pflaster über die
Schnittwunde.
Gipsbinde
Fußgips
Gipsverband

plastisch, formbar

Formbarkeit

plastic surgery *n*

Having had her face badly damaged in a car accident, she needed plastic surgery.

Schönheitschirurgie, plastische Chirurgie
Da Ihr Gesicht durch einen Autounfall schwer verletzt wurde, war plastische Chirurgie notwendig.

pneumonia *n*
Her aunt died of pneumonia at the age of eighty-four.

Lungenentzündung
Ihre Tante starb mit vierundachtzig Jahren an einer Lungenentzündung.

poison *n*
The doctor injected the antidote to the poison.

Gift
Der Arzt spritzte das Gegenmittel um das Gift zu neutralisieren.

poliomyelitis *n*
Nowadays children are vaccinated against poliomyelitis.

Kinderlähmung
Heutzutage werden Kinder gegen Kinderlähmung geimpft.

pollen *n*
A lot of people are allergic to pollen.
pollen allergy

Pollen
Viele Leute sind allergisch gegen Pollen.
Pollenallergie

polyp *n*
A polyp is a small growth in a mucous membrane.

Polyp
Ein Polyp ist eine kleine Wucherung in der Schleimhaut.

postnatal depression *n*
Some mothers suffer from postnatal depression after giving birth.

Wochenbettpsychose
Einige Mütter leiden unter Wochenbettpsychose, nachdem sie ein Kind zur Welt gebracht haben.

posture *n*
He was given special exercises to correct his posture.

Haltung
Man verschrieb ihm spezielle Übungen, um seine Haltung zu verbessern.

predisposition *n*
Some men have a hereditary predisposition to contract prostata cancer at about the age of fifty.

Veranlagung
Einige Männer haben eine genetische Veranlagung, mit etwa fünfzig an Prostata-Krebs zu erkranken.

pregnancy *n*
The pregnancy test was positive.
pregnant

Schwangerschaft
Der Schwangerschaftstest war positiv.
schwanger

premature *n*
The twins were six weeks premature.

premature birth
premature bleeding

vorzeitig
Die Zwillinge wurden sechs Wochen zu früh geboren.
Frühgeburt
Frühblutung

prenatal *adj*
Do your prenatal exercises!

vorgeburtlich
Machen Sie ihre Schwangerschafts-gymnastik!

---

prenatal care
Prenatal is essential to the health of both mother and child.

Schwangerschaftsvorsorge
Die Schwangerschaftsvorsorge ist für die Gesundheit von Mutter und Kind unentbehrlich.

---

pressure bandage *n*
She applied a pressure bandage to stop the bleeding.

Druckverband
Sie verband die Wunde mit einem Druckverband, um das Bluten zu stillen.

---

preventive medicine *n*
Preventive medicine includes testing for specific diseases in order to effect an early cure.

Vorsorgemedizin
Die Vorsorgemedizin schließt das Testen spezifischer Krankheiten ein, um eine frühzeitige Heilung zu bewirken.

---

prickling feeling *n*
She felt a prickling feeling in her legs.

Kribbelgefühl
Sie spürte ein Kribbelgefühl in den Beinen.

---

private *adj*
private patient
She was a private patient in the private ward of a Munich hospital.

privat, Privat-
Privatpatient
Sie war Privatpatientin auf der Privat-station eines Münchener Krankenhauses.

---

probability *n*
The probability of children inheriting certain diseases can be estimated.

Wahrscheinlichkeit
Die Wahrscheinlichkeit, dass Kinder gewisse Krankheiten erben könnten, kann eingeschätzt werden.

---

progesterone *n*
The contraceptive pill contains progesterone.

Gestagen
Die Antibabypille enthält Gestagen.

---

prognosis *n*
The prognosis is not very optimistic.

Prognose
Die Prognose ist nicht sehr optimistisch.

---

prolapse *n*
We speak of a "prolapse", when an organ sinks below its normal position, an example of this being a prolapsed uterus.

Vorfall
Wir reden von einem „Vorfall", wenn ein Organ unter seine normale Position sinkt; ein Beispiel dafür ist die Senkung der Gebärmutter.

---

proliferate *v*

Viruses proliferate under favourable conditions.

sich verbreiten, sich vermehren, wuchern
Viren verbreiten sich in einer günstigen Umgebung.

prophylactic *adj*
One prophylactic measure is teeth-cleaning.
prophylactic inoculation
prophylaxis

Schutz-
Das Zähneputzen ist eine Schutzmaß-nahme.
Schutzimpfung
Prophylaxe, Vorbeugung

---

prostate gland *n*
prostatism
Prostatism occurs through compression or obstruction of the urethra by an enlarged prostate gland, causing difficulty in urination.

Prostata
Prostatismus
Prostatismus wird durch das Ausüben von Druck oder Blockieren der Harnleiter durch eine vergrößerte Prostata ausgelöst und verursacht Schwierigkeiten beim Urinieren.

---

protein *n*
Meat, fish and eggs are high in protein.

Eiweiß
Fleisch, Fisch und Eier haben einen hohen Eiweißgehalt.

---

protruding *adj*
He had a protruding upper lip.

hervortretend
Seine Oberlippe trat hervor.

---

psychiatry *n*
psychiatrist
A psychiatrist treats patients with mental disorders.

Psychiatrie
Psychiater
Ein Psychiater behandelt Patienten, die psychisch krank sind.

---

psychology *n*

Psychology

Some confusion may occur concerning the English word **"psychological"**, which can either be translated as German "psychisch", referring to a mental state, or as "psychologisch", referring to the science of psychology.

---

psychological

psychisch

---

puberty *n*
The hormonal changes which take place during puberty are responsible for the typical pubescent symptoms.

Pubertät
Der Hormonzustand, der während der Pubertät eintritt, ist für die typischen Symptome verantwortlich.

---

pubic hair *n*
In some cultures women remove pubic hair.

Schamhaar
In einigen Kulturen entfernen Frauen ihr Schamhaar.

---

public health *n*
The public health organisation is responsible for standards of hygiene in public places.

öffentliches Gesundheitswesen
Das öffentliche Gesundheitswesen ist für Hygiene-Normen an öffentlichen Orten zuständig.

pulmonary *adj*
The patient was undergoing treatment for pulmonary tuberculosis.

pulse *n*
His pulse was very weak.

pulse rate *n*

pupil *n*
Our pupils dilate in the dark.

pulmonal
Der Patient wurde wegen einer pulmonalen Tuberkulose behandelt.

Puls
Sein Puls war sehr schwach.

Pulsfrequenz

Pupille
Die Pupillen erweitern sich im Dunkeln.

Q/R

quarantine *n*
The length of time a person or animal is kept in quarantine, is calculated as the maximum incubation period of the disease in question.

quiver *v*
He was quivering with fear.

radiography *n*
Radiography is the production of "photographs" (radiographs) using X-rays or gamma rays.

radiotherapy *n*
Radiotherapy is the treatment of disease using radiation.

reflex *n*
They tested his reflexes.
reflex action

regenerate *v*
Recent discoveries have indicated that brain cells can be regenerated.

regress *v*
regression

Regression to childish behaviour makes it possible for patients to avoid anxiety.

Quarantäne
Die Dauer der Quarantäne für Person oder Tier wird nach der Inkubationszeit der in Frage kommenden Krankheit bemessen.

zittern
Er zitterte vor Angst.

Radiographie
In der Radiographie erzeugt man Bilder anhand von Röntgen- oder Gammastrahlen.

Radiotherapie, Strahlentherapie
Radiotherapie ist der Einsatz von Radiation (Strahlung) als Heilmittel.

Reflex
Man überprüfte seine Reflexe.
Reflexhandlung

regenerieren
Neue Entdeckungen zeigen, dass sich Gehirnzellen regenerieren können.

zurückkehren
Rückkehr – in der Psychologie zum kindlichen Verhalten
Die Rückkehr zum kindlichen Verhalten ermöglicht Patienten, sich Sorgen zu entziehen.

regurgitation *n*
regurgitate
Some animals and birds regurgitate semi-digested food to feed their young.

Blood regurgitates when it flows backwards due to a defective valve.

Rückfluss
zurückfließen
Einige Tiere und Vögel füttern ihren Nachwuchs mit teilweise verdauter Nahrung.
Blut kann aufgrund einer defektiven Klappe zurückfließen.

rehabilitation *n*
rehabilitation centre
The ex-drug addict had spent several months in a rehabilitation centre.

Rehabilitation
Rehabilitationszentrum
Der frühere Drogenabhängige hatte einige Monate in einem Rehabilitations-zentrum verbracht.

relapse *n*
His condition had improved, when he suddenly had a relapse.

Rückfall
Sein Zustand hatte sich gerade verbessert, als er plötzlich einen Rückfall erlitt.

relief *n*
It was a relief to hear that she would live.

Erleichterung
Es war eine Erleichterung, zu hören, dass sie leben würde.

relieve *v*
The medicine should relieve the symptoms.

lindern
Die Medizin sollte die Symptome lindern.

remedy *n*
Do you know a good remedy for a sore throat?

Heilmittel
Kennst du ein gutes Heilmittel gegen Halsweh?

remission *n*
If they are lucky, leukaemia patients can enjoy a phase of remission.

Remission
Wenn sie Glück haben, können Leukä-mie-Patienten eine Remissionsphase erleben.

reproduction *n*
Children are taught about sexual reproduction in animals and humans at school.
reproductive organ

Fortpflanzung
Kinder lernen über die Fortpflanzung von Tier und Mensch in der Schule.

Fortpflanzungsorgan

research *n*
research institute
The Max Planck Institutes are famous research institutes in Germany.

Forschung
Forschungsinstitut
Die Max-Planck-Institute sind berühmte Forschungsinstitute in Deutschland.

residue *n*
Chemical analysis is performed on the residue of boiled samples.

Rückstand
Die Rückstände gekochter Proben werden chemisch analysiert.

resistant *adj*
The current flu virus is resistant to several types of antibiotic.

widerstandsfähig, resistent
Der aktuelle Grippevirus ist gegen einige Arten von Antibiotika widerstandsfähig.

respiration *n*
Respiration is the act of taking in oxygen and expiring carbon dioxide.

Atmung
Atmung ist die Aufnahme von Sauerstoff mit gleichzeitiger Abgabe von Kohlendioxid.

respond *v*
The disease responds to treatment.

responsiveness

ansprechen
Der Patient sprach auf die Behandlung gegen seine Krankheit an.
Ansprechbarkeit

rest *n*
The doctor prescribed three tablets a day after meals, and lots of rest.

Ruhe
Der Arzt verschrieb drei Tabletten am Tag nach den Mahlzeiten und viel Ruhe.

resuscitation *n*
resuscitate
They were able to resuscitate him.

Wiederbelebung
wiederbeleben
Man konnte ihn wiederbeleben.

retarded *adj*
The retarded ten year old had a mental age of three.

zurückgeblieben
Das zurückgebliebene Kind stand auf einem geistigen Alter von drei Jahren.

retch *v*
Retching is an involuntary spasm of vomiting.

würgen
Würgen ist ein unwillkürlicher Brechreiz.

retina *n*
The retina is the part of the eye which transmits images to the brain.

Netzhaut
Die Netzhaut ist der Bestandteil des Auges, wodurch Bilder an das Gehirn übermittelt werden.

Rhesus factor n

Rhesusfaktor

The **Rhesus factor** is an agglutinogen first discovered in a rhesus monkey, hence the name. Its presence in human blood – referred to as "Rh positive" – can cause a reaction during pregnancy, or after a blood transfusion, if blood is given which does not contain this factor (Rh negative).

rheumatism *n*
Rheumatism can be very painful, especially in the joints.

Rheumatismus
Rheumatismus kann sehr schmerzhaft sein, besonders in den Gelenken.

rib *n*
The drunken driver was lucky to escape

Rippe
Der betrunkene Autofahrer hatte Glück,

with three fractured ribs when he drove his car into a tree – the accident could have been fatal.

mit drei gebrochenen Rippen davonge-kommen zu sein, als er an einen Baum fuhr – der Unfall hätte tödlich sein können.

rickets n
Rickets used to be common in areas with little sunlight in winter.

Rachitis
Rachitis kam früher in Gebieten mit wenig Sonnenlicht im Winter häufig vor.

rinse (out) v
The dental assistant asked if he would like to rinse out his mouth.

ausspülen
Die Zahnarzthelferin fragte, ob er gerne sein Mund ausspülen würde.

rise v
When his temperature rose, we decided to call the doctor.

ansteigen
Als seine Temperatur anstieg, entschlossen wir, den Arzt zu rufen.

risk of infection n
The school was closed for three weeks due to risk of infection.

Ansteckungsgefahr
Die Schule wurde drei Wochen lang wegen Ansteckungsgefahr geschlossen.

roleplaying n
Roleplaying is a method employed in psychology and teaching.

Rollenspielen
Das Rollenspiel ist eine in der Psychologie und im Unterricht eingesetzte Methode.

S

safe adj
If used according to the instructions, this product is safe.

unbedenklich, sicher
Bei Beachtung der Anleitung ist die Verwendung dieses Produktes unbe-denklich.

saline solution n
Try gargling with a saline solution.

Kochsalzlösung
Probieren Sie mit einer Kochsalzlösung zu gurgeln.

saliva n

Speichel

salmonella n
Food poisoning from salmonella bacteria can result from incorrect storage of food products.

Salmonella
Lebensmittelvergiftung aufgrund Salmo-nella-Bakterien, kann auf die falsche Lagerung von Lebensmitteln zurück-geführt werden.

salt depletion n
People exposed to very hot climates can suffer salt depletion.

Salzmangel
Wer einem sehr heißen Klima ausgesetzt wird, kann an Salzmangel leiden.

sample *n*
The sample was sent to the laboratory.

Probe
Die Probe wurde an das Labor verschickt.

sanatorium *n*
The patient in the sanatorium was chronically ill.
sanatorium therapy

Sanatorium
Der Patient im Sanatorium war chronisch krank.
Sanatoriumsbehandlung

sane *adj*
We considered him to be a sane, well-balanced person.

zurechnungsfähig
Wir hielten ihn für einen zurechnungs-fähigen, ausgeglichenen Menschen.

sanitary *adj*
sanitary towel
The hospital provides sanitary towels.

sanitation

sanitary, hygienisch
Damenbinde
Das Krankenhaus stellt Damenbinden zur Verfügung.
Gesundheitspflege

scab *n*
There was a thick scab on the wound.

Schorf
Es war ein dicker Schorf auf der Wunde.

scald *v*
He scalded his hand on the teapot.

verbrühen
Er verbrühte sich die Hand an der Teekanne.

scale *v*
His teeth were scaled and cleaned.

Zahnstein entfernen
Der Zahnstein wurde entfernt und die Zähne gereinigt.

scalp *n*
He washed his hair and massaged his scalp.

Kopfhaut
Er wusch sich die Haare und massierte die Kopfhaut.

scalpel *n*
A surgeon uses a scalpel.

Skalpell
Ein Chirurg verwendet ein Skalpell.

scanner *n*
A scanner provides an image of an internal organ for diagnostic purposes.
scanning electron microscope

Scanner
Ein Scanner zeigt das Bild eines internen Organs zu diagnostischen Zwecken.
Rasterelektronmikroskop

scar *n*
He had a long scar on his face from a childhood injury.

scar tissue

Narbe
Er hatte eine lange Narbe im Gesicht – das Ergebnis einer Verletzung aus der Kindheit.
Narbengewebe

scared *adj*
She was scared of heights.

verängstigt
Sie hatte Höhenangst.

scarlet fever *n*
The Kindergarten was closed due to an epidemic of scarlet fever.

Scharlach
Der Kindergarten wurde wegen einer Scharlachepidemie geschlossen.

schizophrenic *adj*
His behaviour was diagnosed as schizophrenic.

schizophren
Man stellte fest, sein Verhalten sei schizophren.

sciatica *n*
Sciatica generally refers to pain occurring along the sciatic nerve.

Ischiassyndrom
Das Ischiassyndrom bezieht sich allgemein auf Schmerzen entlang des Ischiasnervs.

science *n*
There are many branches of medical science.

Wissenschaft
Es gibt viele Branchen in der Medizin.

scissors n pl
Can you pass me the scissors, please?

Schere
Kannst du mir bitte die Schere reichen?

scratch *v*
The cat scratched her during the visit to the vet.

kratzen
Die Katze kratzte sie während des Tierarztbesuches.

scrotum *n*
The scrotum contains the testicles.

Hodensack
Die Hoden befinden sich im Hodensack.

scurvy *n*
Sailors used to suffer from scurvy.

Skorbut
Matrosen litten an Skorbut.

seasick *adj*
I was seasick on the ferry from Calais to Dover.

seekrank
Ich war seekrank auf der Fähre von Calais nach Dover.

sebum *n*
Sebum is secreted by the sebaceous glands and ...

Talg
Talg wird von den Talgdrüsen und ...

secrete *v*
... insulin is secreted by the pancreas.

absondern, ausscheiden
... Insulin von der Bauchspeicheldrüse abgesondert.

sedative *n*
The doctor gave the patient a sedative.

Beruhigungsmittel
Der Arzt gab dem Patienten ein Beruhigungsmittel.

sedentary *adj*
People who have sedentary occupations should do plenty of exercise in their free time.

sedentary
Leute, die sedentäre Berufe ausüben, sollten sich in ihrer Freizeit viel bewegen.

self-help group *n*
He was a member of a self-help group.

Selbsthilfegruppe
Er war Mitglied einer Selbsthilfegruppe.

self-treatment *n*
Self-treatment should be restricted to a few days; if the symptoms do not clear up by then, you should see a doctor.

Eigenbehandlung
Eigenbehandlung soll auf ein paar Tage eingeschränkt werden; wenn keine Besserung eingetreten ist, sollten Sie einen Arzt aufsuchen.

senile *adj*
The eighty year old woman was becoming senile – she forgot things more and more frequently.
senilism

senil
Die achtzigjährige Frau wurde senil – sie vergaß Dinge immer öfter.

vorzeitiges Altern

senile cataract *n*
The English pensioner came to Germany for a (senile) cataract operation.
senile debility
senile deafness
senile kerstosis
Cosmetic products claim to be effective against the typical brown marks of senile kerstosis.

Altersstar
Der englische Rentner kam für eine Altersstaroperation nach Deutschland.
Altersschwäche
Altersschwerhörigkeit
Altersflecken
Hersteller kosmetischer Produkte behaupten, dass diese gegen die typischen braunen Altersflecken wirksam einschreiten können.

sensation *n*
The patient complained of a sensation of fullness after meals.
sensation of pressure

Gefühl
Der Patient klagte über Völlegefühl nach den Mahlzeiten.
Druckgefühl

sensitive *adj*
Her skin was very sensitive.
She was a very sensitive person.
sensitivity

sensibel, empfindlich
Ihre Haut war äußerst empfindlich.
Sie war eine sehr sensible Person.
Sensibilität, Empfindlichkeit

septum *n*
A septum divides two cavities or tissues.

Scheidewand
Eine Scheidewand trennt zwei Höhlen oder Gewebe.

severe *adj*
She was severely disabled.
severe trauma

schwerwiegend, schwer
Sie war schwerbehindert.
schweres Trauma

sexual drive *n*
sexual intercourse
The gynaecologist asked her if she had had sexual intercourse.
sexual maturity

Sexualtrieb, Geschlechtstrieb
Geschlechtsverkehr
Der Frauenarzt fragte, ob sie Geschlechtsverkehr gehabt hatte.
Geschlechtsreife

sheet *n*
The nurse changed the sheets.

Laken, Bettlaken
Die Krankenschwester wechselte die Bettlaken.

shift *n*
She was working on the night shift last week.
shift work

Schicht
Sie hatte letzte Woche Nachtdienst.

Schichtarbeit

shinbone *n*
The tibia is referred to in everyday language as the "shinbone".

Schienbein
Im normalen Sprachgebrauch verwendet man „Schienbein" anstatt der lateinischen Bezeichnung „Tibia".

shingles *n*
Shingles is a viral disease.

Gürtelrose
Gürtelrose wird durch einen Virus verursacht.

shock *n*
The passenger was treated for shock.

Schock
Der Fahrgast wurde wegen Schock behandelt.

shortage *n*
British hospitals are experiencing a shortage of nursing staff.

Mangel
Es besteht in britischen Krankenhäusern ein Mangel an Pflegepersonal.

shortness of breath *n*
He was short of breath by the time he reached the fifth floor.

Kurzatmigkeit
Er war kurzatmig, als er das fünfte Stockwerk erreichte.

shortsighted *adj*
She realised she was shortsighted, when she could not read the blackboard from the back row.

kurzsichtig
Ihr wurde klar, dass sie kurzsichtig war, als sie die Tafel von der hinteren Reihe nicht lesen konnte.

short-term memory *n*
My uncle had a very good short-term memory.

Kurzzeitgedächtnis
Mein Onkel hatte ein sehr gutes Kurzzeitgedächtnis.

shoulder *n*
His shoulders were always stiff after sitting at the computer for too long.
shoulder blade
shoulder girdle
shoulder joint

Schulter
Seine Schultern waren immer steif, wenn er zu lange am Computer gesessen hatte.
Schulterblatt
Schultergürtel
Schultergelenk

Siamese twins *n, pl*
The surgeon operated on the Siamese twins to separate them.

siamesische Zwillinge
Der Chirurg operierte die siamesischen Zwillinge, um sie zu trennen.

sick bed *n*
He was lying in his sick bed ...

Krankenbett
Er lag in seinem Krankenbett ...

sick benefit *n*
... and applied for sick benefit, ...

Krankengeld
... und stellte einen Antrag auf Krankengeld, ...

sick leave *n*
... but the doctor only granted him one week's sick leave.

Krankschreibung
... aber der Arzt schrieb ihn nur eine Woche lang krank.

side effects n pl
The drug has no known side-effects.

Nebenwirkungen
Bei diesem Mittel sind keine Nebenwirkungen bekannt.

sign language *n*
The deaf-and-dumb communicate using sign language.

Zeichensprache
Die Taubstummen kommunizieren mittels Zeichensprache.

similarity *n*
There was no similarity between the two cases.

Ähnlichkeit
Es gab keine Ähnlichkeit zwischen den beiden Fällen.

sinusitis *n*
Sinusitis is the inflammation of the membrane which lines the nasal sinus.

Sinusitis
Sinusitis ist eine Nasennebenhöhlenentzündung.

skin *n*
The skin has, among others, protective, excretive and sensory functions.

skin colour
skin disease
skin rash

Haut
Funktionen der Haut sind unter anderem Schutz und Ausscheidung; sie dient auch als Sinnesorgan.
Hautfarbe
Hautkrankheit
Hautausschlag

skull *n*
His skull was injured in the car accident.

skull cap

Schädel
Sein Schädel wurde bei dem Autounfall verletzt.
Schädeldecke

sleep *v*
The patient could not sleep.
sleep
sleeping pill
sleeping sickness

schlafen
Der Patient konnte nicht schlafen.
Schlaf
Schlaftablette
Schlafkrankheit

slightly injured *adj*
He was lucky to be only slightly injured after a bad fall.

leicht verletzt
Er hatte Glück, nach einem schweren Sturz nur leicht verletzt zu sein.

slim *adj* *The patient was a tall, slim girl of nineteen.*	schlank *Die Patientin war eine große, schlanke Frau von neunzehn Jahren.*
slimming cure *n* *Slimming cures often have only a short-lived effect; the pounds soon return.*	Abmagerungskur, Schlankheitskur *Schlankheitskuren haben oft nur eine kurze Wirkung, die Pfunde kehren bald zurück.*
slipped disc *n* *He was in bed with a slipped disc.*	Bandscheibenvorfall *Er lag wegen eines Bandscheibenvorfalls im Bett.*
small intestine *n* *The duodenum is part of the small intestine.*	Dünndarm *Das Duodenum ist Teil des Dünndarms.*
smoker's cough *n*	Raucherhusten

Some illnesses which often result from smoking are named accordingly, for example, **"smoker's cough"** and "smoker's leg".

sneeze *v* *When you have a cold, you sneeze more often than usual.*	niesen *Wenn man erkältet ist, niest man öfter als sonst.*
snore *v* *Her husband snored loudly all night long, so she begged him to see his doctor.*	schnarchen *Ihr Ehemann schnarchte die ganze Nacht lang ziemlich laut; so flehte sie ihn an, seinen Arzt aufzusuchen.*
soluble *adj* *These aspirins are soluble in water.*	löslich *Diese Aspirintabletten lösen sich in Wasser auf.*
sore *adj* *She had a sore throat.*	wund *Sie hatte Halsschmerzen.*
spastic *adj* *Spastic people suffer from spasms and convulsions.*	spastisch *Spastiker leiden unter Anfällen und Schüttelkrämpfen.*
specimen *n* *The specimen was sent to the laboratory for testing.*	Probe *Die Probe wurde zur Untersuchung ins Labor geschickt.*

spectacles *n, pl*
Do you wear spectacles?

Brille
Trägst du eine Brille?

sperm *n*
The student donated sperm.
sperm bank
spermatic duct

Samen
Der Student spendete Samen.
Samenbank
Samenleiter

spina bifida *n*
Spina bifida is a congenital disease.

Spina Bifida
*Spina Bifida ist eine genetische
Krankheit.*

spine *n*

Rückgrat, Wirbelsäule

The **spine**, or spinal column, surrounds the spinal canal. This contains the spinal cord, consisting of nerve tissue, which, together with the brain, forms the central nervous system.

spleen *n*
*One of the functions of the spleen is the
production of antibodies.*

Milz
*Eine Funktion der Milz ist die Produktion
von Antikörpern.*

splint *n*
They put his leg in splints.

Schiene
Sie schienten sein Bein.

sprain *v*
She sprained her ankle.
sprain

verstauchen
Sie verstauchte sich das Fußgelenk.
Verstauchung

spread *v*
*The epidemic spread to the surrounding
villages.*

verbreiten
*Die Epidemie verbreitete sich über die
naheliegenden Dörfer.*

squint *v*
The little girl squinted.

schielen
Das kleine Mädchen schielte.

stabilise *v*
His condition stabilised.

stabilisieren
Sein Zustand stabilisierte sich.

stagger *v*
*The elderly lady staggered into her
apartment; four days later the police
found her body.*

wanken
*Die ältere Frau wankte in ihre Wohnung;
vier Tage später fand die Polizei ihre
Leiche.*

stammer *v*
*The little boy had to go to a speech
therapist because he stammered.*

stammeln
*Der kleine Junge musste zum Logopäden,
weil er stammelte.*

starve *v*
Large numbers of the population of Afghanistan are starving.

verhungern
Viele Menschen in Afghanistan verhungern.

sterile *adj*
She put a sterile dressing on the wound.

steril
Sie legte einen sterilen Verband auf die Wunde.

sterilise *v*
Babies' bottles need to be sterilised.
sterilization

sterilisieren
Babyflaschen müssen sterilisiert werden.
Sterilisation

sternum *n*
The upper seven ribs are attached to the sternum.

Brustbein
Die oberen sieben Rippen sind mit dem Brustbein verbunden.

stethoscope *n*
The GP took his stethoscope out of his bag.

Hörrohr
Der Hausarzt nahm sein Hörrohr aus der Tasche.

stiff *n*
Her joints were stiff.

steif, ungelenkig
Ihre Gelenke waren steif.

stillbirth *n*
stillborn
The baby was stillborn.

Totgeburt
tot geboren
Das Baby wurde tot geboren.

stitch (up) *v*
The surgeon stitched up the wound after operating.

nähen, vernähen
Der Chirurg nähte die Wunde nach der Operation zu.

stomach *n*
stomach pump
A stomach pump is used, after someone has swallowed an overdose of sleeping pills.

Magen
Magenpumpe
Man benutzt eine Magenpumpe, wenn jemand eine Überdosis an Schlaftabletten genommen hat.

stool *n*
The stool specimen was examined, and the results sent to the GP.

Stuhl
Die Stuhlprobe wurde untersucht und die Ergebnisse dem Hausarzt zugeschickt.

stress *n*
A lot of working hours are lost due to stress.
stress factor

Stress
Viele Arbeitsstunden gehen aufgrund von Stress verloren.
Stressfaktor

stretcher *n*
They put the victim of the skiing accident on a stretcher.

Krankentrage
Sie legten das Opfer des Skiunfalls auf eine Krankentrage.

stretchmarks *n, pl*
Massaging with oil during pregnancy helps prevent stretchmarks.

Schwangerschaftsstreifen
Ölmassagen während der Schwangerschaft helfen, Schwangerschaftsstreifen vorzubeugen.

---

stroke *n*
His left side was paralysed after a stroke.

Schlaganfall
Seine linke Seite war nach einem Schlaganfall gelähmt.

---

subconscious *n*
Some memories were present in his subconscious.

Unterbewusstsein
Einige Erinnerungen waren in seinem Unterbewusstsein vorhanden.

---

sucking reflex *n*
The sucking reflex causes a newborn baby to start sucking when it is offered the breast.

Saugreflex
Wegen des Saugreflexes fängt ein Neugeborenes an zu saugen, wenn man es an die Brust legt.

---

suffocate *v*
suffocation
One does not give babies a pillow because of the danger of suffocation.

ersticken
Erstickung
Man gibt Babys wegen hoher Erstickungsgefahr kein Kissen.

---

suicide *n*
He attempted suicide, but the doctors were able to save him.
suicidal

Selbstmord
Er versuchte sich umzubringen, aber die Ärzte konnten ihn retten.
selbstmörderisch

---

sunstroke *n*
He had a sunstroke after foolishly sunbathing for three hours on an Italian beach.

Sonnenstich
Er hatte einen Sonnenstich, nachdem er unvorsichtigerweise drei Stunden lang an einem italienischen Strand in der Sonne lag.

---

suppress *v*
He suppressed his anxiety about his future.

unterdrücken
Er unterdrückte seine Zukunftsangst.

---

surgeon *n*
He is a famous surgeon.
surgical

Chirurg
Er ist ein berühmter Chirurg.
chirurgisch

---

survive *v*
Only three people survived the train crash.

überleben
Nur drei Leute überlebten den Zugunfall.

---

suture *n*
to part a suture
to suture

Naht
eine Naht eröffnen
eine Wunde nähen

sweat *v*
After riding his bicycle three miles to the hospital, he was sweating.

schwitzen
Nachdem er drei Meilen mit dem Rad zum Krankenhaus gefahren war, schwitzte er.

swelling *n*
swollen
Her legs were often swollen at the end of the day.

Schwellung, Anschwellung
geschwollen
Sie hatte am Ende des Tages oft geschwollene Beine.

symptom *n*
Two of the symptoms of a cold are sneezing and a runny nose.

Symptom
Zwei Symptome einer Erkältung: man niest und die Nase läuft.

syndrome *n*
Mongolism is also referred to as Down's syndrome.

Syndrom
Mongolismus wird auch als Down-Syndrom bezeichnet.

syphilis *n*
Syphilis is a venereal disease.

Syphilis
Syphilis ist eine Geschlechtskrankheit.

syringe *n*
The nurse came into my room with a syringe in her hand.

Spritze
Die Krankenschwester kam in mein Zimmer mit einer Spritze in der Hand.

T

tactile sense *n*
Our tactile sense enables us to distinguish between different surfaces, e.g. rough and smooth.
tactile sensation
tactile sensibility

Tastsinn
Unser Tastsinn ermöglicht uns, zwischen verschiedenen Oberflächen zu unterscheiden, z. B. rauhen und glatten.
Berührungsempfindung
Tastempfindlichkeit

tampon *n*
to plug with a tampon

Tampon
mit einem Tampon ausstopfen

tantrum *n*
Toddlers often throw tantrums.

Wutanfall
Kleinkinder haben oft Wutanfälle.

tapeworm *n*
Cats and dogs can have tapeworms.

Bandwurm
Hunde und Katzen können Bandwürmer haben.

tar *n*
Low-tar cigarettes are available.

Teer
Es gibt Zigaretten mit niedrigem Teergehalt.

tattooing *n*
Tattooing became fashionable several years ago.

Tätowierung
Tätowierungen wurden vor einigen Jahren modern.

tea *n*

Tee

The English cure for all problems is a good, strong cup of black **tea,** with milk and sometimes sugar. Whether a mother has just given birth, someone has died, or there is a natural catastrophe, the first thing to do is to put the kettle on.

teaching hospital *n*
She got a job at one of the big teaching hospitals in London.

Ausbildungskrankenhaus
Sie bekam eine Stelle an einem der großen Londoner Ausbildungskrankenhäuser.

tear *n*
We shed tears when we cry.
tear sac

Träne
Die Tränen fließen, wenn wir weinen.
Tränensack

technical term *n*
Technical terms are often derived from Latin.

Fachausdruck
Fachausdrücke stammen oft aus dem Lateinischen.

teeth *n pl*
Clean your teeth after meals!

teething

Zähne
Putzen Sie die Zähne nach den Mahlzeiten!
Zahnen

teetotalism *n*
teetotal
My mother is strictly teetotal.

Abstinenz vom Alkohol
auf Alkohol verzichtend
Meine Mutter trinkt keinen Alkohol.

telepathy *n*
telepathic
Perhaps we are in telepathic communication.

Telepathie
telepathisch
Vielleicht kommunizieren wir telepathisch.

temperature *n*

Temperatur

The word, **temperature,** is often used somewhat inaccurately in English, with the meaning of a "high temperature". We say of someone, "He's got a temperature", when we mean he has a fever.

tendon *n*
A tendon is the connection between a muscle and a bone.

Sehne
Eine Sehne verbindet einen Muskel mit einem Knochen.

tennis elbow *n*
Playing too much tennis can cause inflammation of the elbow, which is then referred to as "tennis elbow".

Tennisarm
Wenn man zu viel Tennis spielt, kann sich der Ellbogen entzünden: diese Entzündung wird dann als „Tennisarm" bezeichnet.

thrombocyte *n*
Platelets are also referred to as thrombocytes.
thrombosis

Thrombozyt
Plättchen werden auch als Thrombozyten bezeichnet.
Thrombose

thumb *n*
The three-year old was always sucking his thumb.
thumb-sucking

Daumen
Der dreijährige Junge lutschte immer am Daumen.
Daumenlutschen

thyroid *n*
The thyroid gland can be over and underactive.
thyroid hormone

Schilddrüse
Es kann sowohl eine Über- als auch eine Unterfunktion der Schilddrüse entstehen.
Schilddrüsenhormon

tibia *n*
He fractured his tibia.

Schienbein
Er hat sich das Schienbein gebrochen.

tick *n*
There are ticks in the Bavarian forests.

tick-borne encephalitis

Zecke
Es gibt Zecken in den bayerischen Wäldern.
Zeckenenzephalitis

tincture *n*
A tincture is an alcohol solution containing a medicinal substance.
tincture of iodine

Tinktur
Eine Tinktur ist die Auflösung eines medizinischen Stoffes in Alkohol.
Jodtinktur

tissue *n*
Tissue is the word used to describe connective living cells.

Gewebe
„Gewebe" beschreibt eine Zusammensetzung von lebenden Zellen.

toe *n*
Humans have ten toes.
toenail

Zehe
Menschen haben zehn Zehen.
Zehnagel

tomogram *n*
tomography
Tomography provides cross-section X-rays of the body.

Tomogramm
Tomographie
Tomographie ermöglicht Querschnittsröntgenbilder des Körpers.

tonic *n*
What you need is a good tonic!

Tonikum
Was Sie brauchen, ist ein gutes Tonikum!

tonsil *n*
tonsillitis
She was at home from school for two weeks with tonsillitis.

tooth *n*
The dentist replaced a filling in my tooth.

toothache

torn ligament *n*
He tore a ligament.

tourniquet *n*
He applied a tourniquet to the upper arm to stop the bleeding.

toxemia *n*
Toxemia is a condition caused by the presence of toxins in the blood.

toxic *adj*
This product is non-toxic.
toxicology

trachea *n*
tracheoscopy
tracheotomy
A tracheotomy is performed when air can no longer reach the lungs due to a blockage.

tract *n*
The alimentary canal is the digestive tract.

traditional medicine *n*
There are a variety of alternatives to traditional medicine.

transfusion *n*
People are given a blood transfusion when they have lost a lot of blood.

transplantation *n*
transplant
The heart transplant patient was doing well.

Mandel
Mandelentzündung
Das Schulmädchen war mit einer Mandelentzündung zwei Wochen zu Hause.

Zahn
Der Zahnarzt ersetzte eine Füllung in meinem Zahn.
Zahnschmerzen

Bänderriss
Er hatte einen Bänderriss.

Tourniquet
Er brachte ein Tourniquet am Oberarm an, um die Blutung zu stillen.

Toxämie
Toxämie wird durch die Anwesenheit von toxischen Substanzen im Blut verursacht.

giftig, toxisch
Dieses Produkt ist ungiftig.
Toxikologie

Luftröhre
Tracheoskopie
Luftröhrenschnitt
Ein Luftröhrenschnitt wird durchgeführt, wenn Luft nicht mehr in die Lungen eindringen kann, weil der Luftweg verstopft ist.

Trakt
Der Verdauungskanal heißt auch Verdauungstrakt.

Schulmedizin
Es gibt einige Alternativen zur Schulmedizin.

Transfusion
Menschen, die viel Blut verloren haben, bekommen eine Bluttransfusion.

Transplantation
Transplantat
Dem Patienten mit dem Herztransplantat ging es gut.

transsexual *adj*
Someone who is transsexual has the feeling of belonging to the opposite sex.

transsexuell
Ein transsexueller Mensch fühlt sich dem anderen Geschlecht zugehörig.

trauma *n*
traumatic
Refugees have often had traumatic experiences in their native countries.
traumatic cataract
traumatic fever

Trauma
traumatisch
Asylsuchende hatten oft traumatische Erlebnisse in ihrem Heimatland.
Wundstar
Wundfieber

tremor *n*
Tremor is one of the symptoms of Parkinson's disease.

Tremor, Zittern
Tremor ist ein Symptom der Parkinson-Krankheit.

triplet *m*
She gave birth to triplets.

Drillinge
Sie brachte Drillinge zur Welt.

tropical disease *n*
Malaria is a tropical disease.
tropical medicine

Tropenkrankheit
Malaria ist eine Tropenkrankheit.
Tropenmedizin

tube *n*

Schlauch

Surgeons insert tubes to bypass blockages. However, the word **"tube"** is sometimes used as an abbreviation for the Eustachian or Fallopian tubes. A tubectomy is the surgical removal of the Fallopian tubes.

tuberculosis *n*
The diagnosis of tuberculosis in its early stages prevents the spread of infection.

Tuberkulose
Die Frühdiagnose von Tuberkulose verhindert die Verbreitung der Infektion.

tumour *n*
The surgeon was able to remove the tumour.

Tumor
Der Chirurg konnte den Tumor entfernen.

twins *n pl*
My cousin gave birth to identical twins.

Zwillinge
Meine Kusine brachte eineiige Zwillinge zur Welt.

twitch *v*
twitching
Twitching is an involuntary movement.

zucken
Zucken
Zucken ist eine unwillkürliche Bewegung.

typhoid fever *n*
Typhoid fever can be contracted by drinking contaminated water.

Typhus
Man kann durch das Trinken infizierten Wassers an Typhus erkranken.

U

ulcer *n*
He was having treatment for a stomach ulcer.
ulcer haemorrhage
ulceration

Geschwür
Er wurde wegen eines Magengeschwürs behandelt.
Ulkusblutung
Geschwürbildung

ultrasound examination *n*
I had an appointment for an ultrasound examination.

Ultraschalluntersuchung
Ich hatte einen Termin für eine Ultraschalluntersuchung.

umbilical cord *n*
The umbilical cord connects the foetus with the placenta.
umbilical cord clamp

Nabelschnur
Die Nabelschnur verbindet den Foetus mit der Plazenta.
Nabelschnurklemme

umbilical hernia *n*
Babies sometimes have an umbilical hernia.

Nabelbruch
Babys haben manchmal einen Nabelbruch.

unborn *adj*
They were still thinking about a name for the as yet unborn child.

ungeboren
Sie dachten noch an einem Namen für das ungeborene Kind.

uncomfortable *adj*
She felt very uncomfortable as she sat in the waiting room.
The bed was uncomfortable.

unbehaglich, unbequem
Sie fühlte sich sehr unbehaglich, als sie im Wartezimmer saß.
Das Bett war unbequem.

unconscious *adj*
He was unconscious for nearly half an hour.
unconsciousness

bewusstlos, ohnmächtig
Er war fast eine halbe Stunde bewusstlos.

Bewusstlosigkeit

under age *adj*
Her parents had to sign the forms, because she was under age.

unmündig
Ihre Eltern mussten die Formulare unterschreiben, weil sie unmündig war.

underarm perspiration *n*
Antiperspirants stop underarm perspiration.

Achselschweiß
Antitranspirant-Deodorants verhindern Achselschweiß.

underdeveloped *adj*
The medical facilities need to be improved in some underdeveloped countries.

unterentwickelt
Medizinische Einrichtungen bedürfen einer Verbesserung in manchen unterentwickelten Ländern.

undernourished *adj*
According to the news, many children in Kuwait are undernourished.

unterernährt
In den Nachrichten liest man, dass viele Kinder in Kuwait unterernährt sind.

underweight *adj*
The girl was severely underweight, and suffering from anorexia nervosa.

unter dem Normalgewicht
Ihr Gewicht lag weit unter dem Normalwert und die junge Frau litt an Anorexia Nervosa.

undiluted *adj*
Take the medicine, undiluted, three times a day.

unverdünnt
Nehmen Sie die Medizin unverdünnt dreimal am Tag.

unfit *adj*
The food was unfit for human consumption.

untauglich, ungeeignet
Die Lebensmittel waren für den Verzehr durch Menschen nicht geeignet.

unhealthy *adj*
Fast food is considered unhealthy.

ungesund
Fastfood wird für ungesund gehalten.

unhygienic *adj*
The conditions in the kitchen were simply unhygienic.

unhygienisch
Die Küche war einfach in einem unhygienischen Zustand.

unstable *adj*
His condition was unstable.

instabil
Sein Zustand war instabil.

unwell *adj*
She was feeling unwell.

unwohl
Sie fühlte sich unwohl.

upper arm *n*
She had bruises on both upper arms.

Oberarm
Sie hatte an beiden Oberarmen Prellungen.

urethra *n*
Urine is eliminated from the bladder through the urethra.

Harnröhre
Urin wird von der Blase durch die Harnröhre ausgeschieden.

urge *n*
She felt a continual urge to urinate.

Drang
Sie fühlte einen ununterbrochenen Drang, Wasser zu lassen.

urgent *adj*
The patient was in urgent need of medical attention.

dringend
Der Patient bedarf dringender medizinischer Hilfe.

urine *n*
The pregnant woman handed in a urine sample.

Urin
Die schwangere Frau gab eine Urinprobe ab.

urology *n*
urologist
He made an appointment with a urologist.

uterus *n*
A hysterectomy is the removal of the uterus.

V

vaccination n
vaccinate
He is vaccinated against rabies.

vaccine *n*
We hope there will soon be a vaccine available against AIDS.

vagina *n*
vaginal smear
The gynaecologist took a vaginal smear.

vaginoscopy

valerian *n*
Valerian is a useful tranquilizer.

valerian drops

valve *n*
If a valve is defective, the blood can flow backwards.
valve orifice
valvular heart defect

varicose vein *n*
Varicose veins can be a symptom of pregnancy, due to the increased weight the legs have to carry.

vasectomy *n*
Husbands may choose to have a vasectomy, when they feel their family is complete.

Urologie
Urologe
Er machte bei einem Urologen einen Termin aus.

Gebärmutter
Eine Hysterektomie ist die Entfernung der Gebärmutter.

Impfung
impfen
Er ist gegen Tollwut geimpft.

Impfstoff
Wir hoffen, dass es bald ein Impfstoff gegen Aids geben wird.

Scheide
Scheidenabstrich
Der Frauenarzt nahm einen Scheidenabstrich.
Scheidenspiegelung

Baldrian
Baldrian ist ein nützliches Beruhigungsmittel.
Baldriantropfen

Klappe
Sollte eine Klappe defekt sein, kann das Blut rückwärts fließen.
Klappenöffnung
Herzklappenfehler

Krampfader
Krampfadern können ein Symptom der Schwangerschaft sein, aufgrund des zusätzlichen, von den Beinen zu tragenden, Gewichts.

Samenleiterdurchtrennung
Ehemänner entscheiden vielleicht, eine Samenleiterdurchtrennung durchführen zu lassen, wenn sie das Gefühl haben, ihre Familie sei komplett.

vegetarian *n*
vegetarian
A vegetarian diet is said to be healthier than one which includes meat.

Vegetarier
vegetarisch
Eine vegetarische Diät soll gesünder sein als eine Diät, die Fleisch enthält.

vein *n*
The veins carry blood containing carbon dioxide back to the lungs from the rest of the body.
vein bypass
vein grafting
vein stripping
venepuncture
venous

Vene
Die Venen transportieren Blut, das Kohlendioxid enthält, vom restlichen Körper zurück zu den Lungen.
Venen-Bypass
Venentransplantation
Venenstripping
Venenpunktion
venös

venereal disease *n*
Syphilis is a serious venereal disease.

Geschlechtskrankheit
Syphilis ist eine ernste Geschlechts-krankheit.

ventilator *n*
A patient who is unable to breathe normally, is attached to a ventilator.

ventilate
ventilatory arrest

Ventilator
Ein Patient, der nicht natürlich atmen kann, wird an einen Ventilator ange-schlossen.
beatmen
Atemstillstand

ventricle *n*
The heart has a left and right ventricle.

Ventrikel
Das Herz hat einen linken und einen rechten Ventrikel.

W

waist *n*
She has a very slim waist.

Taille
Sie hat eine sehr schlanke Taille.

waiting list n

Warteliste

There are long **waiting lists** in Britain for appointments with specialists and routine operations on the National Health Service. Recently some patients have been coming to Germany for private treatment, which is cheaper than in the United Kingdom. This is a serious problem, which the government in Britain will have to resolve.

wake up *v*
Patients in British hospitals are woken up at six o'clock in the morning with a cup of tea.

aufwachen
Patienten in britischen Krankenhäusern werden um sechs Uhr morgens mit einer Tasse Tee geweckt.

walker *n*
I often see elderly people on the streets pushing a walker in front of them as they go.

Gehstütze
Ich sehe oft ältere Leute auf den Straßen, die eine Gehstütze vor sich herschieben.

ward physician *n*
The ward physician was doing his morning round as usual.

Stationsarzt
Der Stationsarzt machte wie üblich seine Vormittagsrunde.

wart *n*
She had several warts on her fingers.

Warze
Sie hatte einige Warzen an den Fingern.

wash down *v*
Swallow the tablet and wash it down with a glass of mineral water.

hinunterspülen
Schlucken Sie die Tablette und spülen Sie sie mit einem Glas Mineralwasser hinunter.

wasp sting *n*
His arm was badly swollen where the wasp had stung him, and the doctor gave him a penicillin injection.

Wespenstich
Sein Arm war dort, wo die Wespe ihn gestochen hatte, sehr geschwollen und der Arzt gab ihm eine Penizillinspritze.

water *n*
Would you like a glass of water?

Wasser
Möchten Sie ein Glas Wasser?

water retention *n*
Water retention may be a problem a few days before a woman's period.

Wassereinlagerung
Wassereinlagerung kann ein paar Tage vor der Periode einer Frau ein Problem sein.

weak *adj*
He was still feeling weak after the operation.
weak eyesight

schwach
Er fühlte sich noch schwach nach der Operation.
Sehschwäche

wean *v*
The baby was weaned at six months.

abstillen
Das Baby wurde mit sechs Monaten abgestillt.

weight *n*
She has lost a lot of weight recently.
weight curve
weight gain
weight loss

Gewicht
Sie hat in letzter Zeit viel abgenommen.
Gewichtskurve
Gewichtszunahme
Gewichtsverlust

well-being *n*
A state of well-being is important in the recovery stage after an illness.

Wohlbefinden
Ein Zustand des Wohlbefindens ist in der Erholungsphase nach einer Krankheit wichtig.

wheelchair *n*
I have a pupil in my class, in a wheelchair.

Rollstuhl
Ich habe eine Rollstuhlfahrerin in meiner Klasse.

whooping cough *n*
For a while, the vaccination against whooping cough was considered unsafe.

Keuchhusten
Für eine Weile wurde die Impfung gegen Keuchhusten für unsicher gehalten.

wisdom tooth *n*
She had to have her wisdom teeth removed.

Weisheitszahn
Sie musste die Weisheitszähne ziehen lassen.

withdrawal symptoms *n, pl*
The heroin addict was experiencing serious withdrawal symptoms.

Entzugserscheinungen
Der Heroinsüchtige litt unter schweren Entzugserscheinungen.

withempty stomach *adj*
Operations are performed on patients with an empty stomach.

nüchtern
Patienten werden bei nüchternem Magen operiert.

X/Y/Z

xerocheilia *n*
My friend suffers from xerocheilia.

Lippentrockenheit
Meine Freundin leidet an Lippentrockenheit.

X-ray *n*
She hasn't seen the X-ray yet.

Röntgenbild
Sie hat das Röntgenbild noch nicht gesehen.

yellow fever *n*
He has to get a vaccination against yellow fever, as he is flying to Africa.

Gelbfieber
Da er nach Afrika fliegt, muss er sich gegen Gelbfieber impfen lassen.

yoke-bone *n*
He fractured his yoke-bone while playing rugby.

Jochbein
Er hat sich beim Rugby das Jochbein gebrochen.

zone therapy *n*
She had to go to the rehabilitation centre for a zone therapy.

Reflexzonentherapie
Sie musste wegen einer Reflexzonentherapie in die Reha.

zoonosis *n*
Rabies is a zoonosis.

Zoonose
Tollwut ist eine Tierkrankheit (Zoonose).

zygote *n*
They implanted the zygote in the uterus.

befruchtete Eizelle
Die befruchtete Eizelle wurde in die Gebärmutter eingesetzt.

A

Abbinden: *ligature*
Abdomen, Unterleib: *abdomen*
Abführmittel: *laxative*
Abhorchen: *auscultate*
Abmagerungskur, Schlankheitskur: *slimming cure*
abschürfen: *graze*
absondern, ausscheiden: *secrete*
Absorption: *absorptio*
aufnehmen, absorbieren: *to absorb*
absaugen: *drain*
abstillen: *wean*
Abstinenz vom Alkohol: *teetotalism*
auf Alkohol verzichtend: *teetotal*
Abstinenz: *abstinence*
Abszess: *abscess*
Abtreibung: *abortion*
Abwehr: *defence*
Achsel: *armpit*
Achselhaar: *axillary hair*
Achselschweiß: *underarm perspiration*
Adamsapfel: *Adam's apple*
Adaptation, Anpassung: *adaptation*
anpassen, sich anpassen: *adapt*
Adrenalin: *adrenalin*
adstringierend: *astringent*
Aggression: *aggression*
aggressiv: *aggressive*
Ähnlichkeit: *similarity*
Akkumulation: *accumulation*
Akne: *acne*
Akupunktur: *acupuncture*
akut: *acute*
Albino: *albino*
Aldehyd: *aldehyde*
alert, rege, aufmerksam: *alert*
Alkohol: *alcohol*
Alkoholiker: *alcoholic*
Alkoholismus: *alcoholism*
Anonyme Alkoholiker: *Alcoholics Anonymous*
allgemeines Befinden: *general condition*
Allgemeinmediziner, Hausarzt: *general practitioner*
Altersflecken: *senile kerstosis*

Altersstar: *senile cataract*
Altersschwäche: *senile debility*
Altersschwerhörigkeit: *senile deafness*
Amalgam: *amalgam*
Ambulanz: *outpatients' department*
Amenorrhoea: *amenorrhoea*
Amnesie, Gedächtnisschwäche, Gedächtnisschwund: *amnesia*
Amöbenruhr: *amoebic dysentery*
Ampulle: *ampoule*
Analgetikum: *analgesic*
Anämie, Blutarmut: *anaemia*
Anamnese: *anamnesis*
Aneurysma: *aneurysm*
Anfall: *attack*
angeborener Geburtsfehler: *congenital defect*
Angina: *angina*
Angina Pectoris: *angina pectoris*
Anorexie: *anorexia*
ansprechen: *respond*
Ansprechbarkeit: *responsiveness*
ansteckend: *contagious*
Ansteckungsgefahr: *risk of infection*
ansteigen: *rise*
Antazidum: *antacid*
Antibiotikum: *antibiotic*
Antidepressivum: *antidepressant*
Antidot, Gegengift: *antidote*
Antihistaminikum: *antihistamine*
Antikoagulans, gerinnungshemmende Substanz: *anticoagulant*
antiseptisch, keimtötend: *antiseptic*
antiseptisch: *antiseptic*
Aphasie: *aphasia*
Apoplexie, Gehirnschlag, Hirnschlag: *apoplexy*
Apotheke: *pharmacy*
Appendix, Blinddarm: *appendix*
Appendizitis: *appendicitis*
Applikator: *applicator*
Armvene: *brachial vein*
Arsen: *arsenic*

Arterie, Schlagader: *artery*
Arteriosklerose: *arteriosclerosis*
Arthritis, Gelenkentzündung:
  arthritis
Arthroskopie: *arthroscopy*
Arzt: *physician*
Ärzteregister: *medical register*
Asthma: *asthma*
Atem, Atemzug: *breath*
Atemnot: *breathlessness*
Atmung: *respiration*
Attest: *medical certificate*
auf Abruf: *on call*
auflösen: *dissolve*
aufschlitzen: *lacerate*
aufwachen: *wake up*
Augenentzündung: *opthalmia*
Augenoptiker: *optician*
ausatmen: *expire*
Ausbildungskrankenhaus: *teaching
  hospital*
Ausfluss: *effluent*
Ausscheidung: *excretion*
ausscheiden: *excrete*
Ausscheidung: *elimination*
ausspülen: *rinse (out)*
Ausstattung, Geräte: *equipment*
Autismus: *autism*
autistisch: *autistic*
Autopsie: *autopsy*
Azidose: *acidosis*

B

Bachblüten: *Bach flowers*
Badezusätze: *bath salts*
Bakterien: *bacteria*
Baldrian: *valerian*
Baldriantropfen: *valerian drops*
Balsam: *balm*
Band: *ligament*
Bänderriss: *torn ligament*
Bandscheibenvorfall: *slipped
  disc*
Bandwurm: *tapeworm*
Bandwurmbefall: *tapeworm
  infestation*
Barbiturat: *barbiturate*
Bartflechte: *barber's rash*
Bartholin-Drüse: *Bartholin's gland*

Bastard: *bastard*
Bauchfellentzündung: *perito-
  nitis*
Bauchhöhlenschwangerschaft: *ecto-
  pic pregnancy*
Bauchnabel: *belly button*
Bauchspeicheldrüse: *pancreas*
Bazillus: *bacillus*
Beckenboden: *pelvic floor*
Becken: *pelvis*
behandelnder Arzt: *attending
  physician*
Behandlungszimmer: *consulting
  room*
behindert: *disabled*
behindert: *handicapped*
Behinderung: *handicap*
benommen: *light headed*
Beruhigungsmittel: *sedative*
Beruhigungsmittel: *calmative*
Beschäftigungstherapie: *occu-
  pational therapy*
Betablocker: *beta-blocker*
Betacarotin: *betacarotene*
Betriebsarzt: *company
  physician*
Betriebsunfall: *industrial
  accident*
betrunken: *intoxicated*
Beutel: *bag*
Beutelwechsel: *bag change
  procedure*
bewusstlos, ohnmächtig: *un-
  conscious*
Bewusstlosigkeit: *unconscious-
  ness*
Bewusstsein: *consciousness*
Bindehautentzündung: *conjunc-
  tiva*
Bindehaut: *conjunctivitis*
Biopsie: *biopsy*
Biotyp: *biotype*
Blähungen: *flatulence*
Blasenentzündung: *cystitis*
Blinddarm: *caecum*
Blinddarmentzündung: *caecitis*
Blinddarmeröffnung: *caecotomy*
Blinddarmkrebs: *caecum cancer*
Blindenschrift: *braille*

Blut: *blood*
Blutbank: *blood bank*
Blutbild: *blood count*
Blutbeutel: *blood pack*
Blutentnahmeset: *blood drawing set*
Blutgruppe: *blood group*
Bluterguss: *bruise*
Blut entnehmen: *draw blood*
Bluterkrankheit: *haemophilia*
Bluthochdruck: *hypertension*
Blutkörperchen: *blood corpuscle*
Blutspender: *blood donor*
Bluttransfusion: *blood transfusion*
Blutgefäße: *blood vessels*
Blutung: *bleeding*
Blutvergiftung: *blood poisoning*
Blutdruck: *blood pressure*
Blutzucker: *blood sugar*
Blutzuckerspiegel: *blood sugar level*
Blutprobe: *blood test*
Bolusinjektion: *bolus injection*
bösartig: *malignant*
Breitband-Antibiotikum: *broad-spectrum antibiotic*
breitschultrig: *broad-shouldered*
Brille: *glasses*
Brille: *spectacles*
Brom: *bromine*
Bronchien: *bronchia*
Bronchiolen: *bronchioles*
Bronchitis: *Bronchitis*
Bronchoskop: *bronchoscope*
Bronchoskopie: *bronchoscopy*
Brustamputation: *mastectomy*
Brustbein: *sternum*
Brustdrüse: *breast*
Brustkrebs: *breast cancer*
Abtasten der Brust: *breast palpitation*
Brustwarze: *nipple*
Brutkasten: *incubator*
Bulimie, Ess-Brechsucht: *bulimia*
Bypass: *bypass*

C

Candidiasis: *candidiasis*
Cerebellum, Kleinhirn: *cerebellum*
Cerumen, Ohrenschmalz: *cerumen*
Chemotherapie: *chemotherapy*
Chirurg: *surgeon*
Chloasma: *chloasma*
Cholera: *cholera*
Cholesterin: *cholesterol*
Chromosom: *chromosome*
chronische Bronchitis: *chronic bronchitis*
Computertomographie: *computerized tomography*
Cortex: *cortex*
Cortex Cerebri: *cerebral cortex*
Cortisol: *cortisol*
Cushing-Krankheit: *Cushing's disease or syndrome*
Cutis, Haut: *cutis*

D

Damenbinde: *sanitary napkin*
Dämmerschlaf: *twilight sleep*
Dämmerungsblindheit: *twilight blindness*
Dammschnitt: *perineotomy*
Dauer-: *long-term*
Dauerbehandlung: *long-term treatment*
Dampfbehandlung: *vapotherapy*
Darm: *bowels*
Darmabführung: *catharsis*
Darmbeschwerden: *intestinal complaints*
Darmblähung: *meteorism*
Darmblutung: *intestinal bleeding*
Darmdrüsen: *intestinal glands*
Darmeinlauf: *enema*
Darmentleerung: *evacuation*
Darmflora: *intestinal flora*
Darmgeschwür: *intestinal ulcer*
Darmgrippe: *intestinal flu*
Dauerheilung: *permanent cure*
Dauerschaden: *permanent damage*
Dauerschmerz: *persistent pain*
Daumen: *thumb*
Daumenlutschen: *thumb-sucking*

Deformierung: *deformation*
Degeneration: *degeneration*
Degenerationskrankheit: *degenerative disease*
Degenerationspsychose: *degenerative psychosis*
degenerieren: *degenerate*
Dehnung: *distention*
Dehydration: *dehydration*
dekalzifizieren: *decalcify*
delirant: *delirious*
Delirium: *delirium*
Deltamuskel: *deltoid muscle*
Demand-Schrittmacher: *demand pacemaker*
den Arzt rufen: *call in a doctor*
Depression: *depression*
Depressivum: *depressant*
deprimiert: *depressed*
Derma: *derma*
Dermatitis: *dermatitis*
Dermatologie: *dermatology*
Dermatologist: *dermatologist*
Desensibilisierung: *desensitisation*
Desoxyribonukleinsäure: *deoxyribonucleic acid*
Diabetes Mellitus: *diabetes mellitus*
Diagnose: *diagnosis*
diagnostizieren: *diagnose*
Dialyse: *dialysis*
Diät: *diet*
diätetisch: *dietary*
dick: *fat*
Dickdarm: *colon*
Diptherie: *diphtheria*
Dismenorrhoe: *dysmenorrhoea*
Doppelkinn: *double chin*
Dosierung: *dosage*
Down-Syndrom: *Down's syndrome*
Dragee: *coated pill*
Drainage: *drainage*
Drang: *urge*
Drillinge: *triplet*
dringend: *urgent*
Droge, Arzneimittel: *drug*
Drogenklinik: *drug clinic*
Druckverband: *pressure bandage*

Drüse: *gland*
Drüsenschwellung: *glandular swelling*
Drüsenerkrankung: *glandular disease*
Drüsenfieber: *glandular fever*
Drüsenfunktion: *glandular function*
Drüsensekret: *glandular secretion*
Dünndarm: *small intestine*
Duodenum, Zwölffingerdarm: *duodenum*
Durchblutungsstörung: *disturbance of circulation*
Durchfall, Diarrhoe: *diarrhoea*
Durchspülung: *washing out*
durchtrennen: *cut*
Dysfunktion: *dysfunction*

E

Echokardiogramm: *echocardiogram*
Echografie: *echography*
EEG – Elektroenzephalogramm: *EEG – electroencephalogram*
Eid des Hippokrates: *Hippocratic oath*
Eierstock: *ovary*
Eigenbehandlung: *self-treatment*
Eileiter: *fallopian tube*
Eingeweide: *intestines*
Einlauf: *enema*
Einlieferung ins Krankenhaus, Aufenthalt im Krankenhaus: *hospitalization*
Einreibemittel: *liniment*
Einschnitt: *incision*
einspritzen: *inject*
Eintrittswunde, Einschuss: *entry wound*
Eisbeutel: *icebag*
Eisenmangel: *iron deficiency*
Eiteransammlung: *accumulation of pus*
eitern: *fester*
Eiweiß: *protein*
Ejakulation: *ejaculation*
EKG – Elektrokardiogramm: *ECG – electrocardiogram*
Ekzem: *eczema*

Elektrochirurgie: *electrosurgery*
Elektrode: *electrode*
Elektrolyse: *electrolysis*
Ellbogen: *elbow*
Embolie: *embolism*
Embryo: *embryo*
Emphysem: *emphysema*
emulgieren: *emulsify*
endokardial: *endocardiac*
Endoskop: *endoscope*
Endoskopie: *endoscopy*
Entbindung: *delivery*
entbinden, zur Welt bringen: *deliver*
Entbindungsstation: *maternity ward*
entgiften: *detoxify*
enthaaren: *depilate*
Enthaarung: *depilation*
entkräften: *debilitate*
entlassen: *discharge*
Entlassungsdiagnose: *diagnosis on discharge*
Entlausung: *delousing*
Entlausungsmittel: *lousicide*
entseuchen: *disinfect*
Entseuchung: *disinfection*
Entschlackung: *purging*
entspannen: *relax*
entwässern: *dry*
Entwässerung: *drying*
Entwicklung: *development*
entwickeln: *develop*
Entwicklungsstörung: *developmental disturbance*
entwurmen: *de-worm*
Entziehungskur: *withdrawal cure*
Entzugserscheinungen: *withdrawal symptoms*
Entzündung: *inflammation*
entzündungshemmend, antiinflammatorisch: *anti-inflammatory*
Enzephalitis: *encephalitis*
Enzym: *enzyme*
Epidemie: *epidemic*
Epidemieherd: *epidemic focus*
Epidermis: *epidermis*
Epiduralanästhesie: *epidural anaesthetic*

Epilepsie: *epilepsy*
Epilepsieanfall: *epileptic fit*
Erbfehler: *genetic defect*
Erbgut: *heritage*
Erbkrankheit: *hereditary disease*
Erektion: *erection*
erfrieren: *freeze to death*
Erfrierung: *frostbite*
Erfrierungstod: *death by exposure*
Erguss: *effusion*
erholen, sich: *recover*
Erkältung: *cold*
Erziehungsurlaub: *maternity leave*
Erleichterung: *relief*
Ernährung: *nutrition*
Ernährung mit der Flasche: *bottle-feeding*
Erschöpfung: *exhaustion*
Erste Hilfe: *first aid*
ersticken: *suffocate*
Erstickung: *suffocation*
ertragen: *endure*
ertrinken: *drown*
Essgewohnheit: *eating habit*
Etikett: *label*
Eustachische Röhre: *Eustachian tube*
Euthanasie: *euthanasia*
Evakuation, Entleerung: *evacuation*
entleeren: *evacuate*

F
Fachausdruck: *technical term*
Familienhintergrund: *family background*
Fango: *fango*
farbenblind: *colour blind*
Fasten, Nulldiät: *fasting*
Fehlbildung: *malformation*
Fehlgeburt: *miscarriage*
Ferse: *heel*
Fersensporn: *heelspur*
Fett: *fat, fatty*
Fettleber: *fatty liver*
Leberverfettung: *fatty metamorphosis of liver*
fettarm: *low-fat*
fettleibig: *obese*

Fettleibigkeit: *obesity*
Fibrose: *fibrosis*
Fieber: *fever*
Fieberdelirium: *delirium*
Fleischwunde: *flesh wound*
Floh: *flea*
Flüssigkeit: *liquid*
Flüssigkeitshaushalt: *fluid balance*
Forschung: *research*
Forschungsinstitut: *research institute*
Fortpflanzung: *reproduction*
Fortpflanzungsorgan: *reproductive organ*
Fötus: *foetus*
Frauenleiden: *female complaint*
fruchtbar: *fertile*
früh: *early*
Frühstadium: *early stage*
Fußpflege: *pedicure*
Fußpilz: *athlete's foot*

G

Galle, Gallenflüssigkeit: *bile*
Gallengang: *biliary duct*
Gallensteine: *gall stones*
Gänsehaut: *goose pimples*
ganzheitlich: *holistic*
Gaumen: *palate*
Gebärmutter: *uterus*
Gebärmutterentfernung: *hysterectomy*
Gebühr, Honorar: *fee*
Geburt bei Steißlage: *breech delivery*
Geburtenkontrolle: *birth control*
Geburtshelfer: *obstetrician*
Geburtsurkunde: *birth certificate*
Gedächtnis: *memory*
Gefahr: *danger*
gefährden: *endanger*
Gefühl: *sensation*
Gegenanzeige: *contraindication*
Gehirn: *brain*
Gehirnerschütterung: *brain concussion*
Gehirnhautentzündung: *meningitis*
Gehirntumor: *brain tumour*

Gehstütze: *walker*
geisteskrank: *insane*
geistig behindert: *mentally handicapped*
Gelbsucht: *jaundice*
Gelenk: *joint*
Gelenkkapsel: *joint capsule*
Gemeinschaftspraxis: *group practice*
Genesung: *convalescence*
genetische Beratung: *genetic counselling*
genital: *genital*
Genitalorgan: *genital organ*
Gentechnologie: *genetic engineering*
Geriatrie: *geriatrics*
geriatrisch: *geriatric*
Gerichtsmedizin: *forensic medicine*
Gerontologie: *gerontology*
Gesäß: *buttocks*
Geschlechtskrankheit: *venereal disease*
geschwollen: *swollen*
Geschwür: *ulcer*
Gestagen: *progesterone*
Gesundheit: *health*
gesund: *healthy*
Gewebe: *tissue*
Gewebeverkalkung: *calcareous degneration*
Gewicht: *weight*
Gewichtszunahme: *weight gain*
Gewichtsverlust: *weight loss*
Gicht: *gout*
Gift: *poison*
giftig, toxisch: *toxic*
Gips, Pflaster: *plaster*
Glaukom: *glaucoma*
Gleichgewicht: *balance*
Gleitmittel: *lubricant*
Glied: *limb*
Glukose: *glucose*
Grad: *degree*
Greifreflex: *grasp reflex*
Grenzlinie: *borderline*

Grippe: *influenza*
Größenwahn: *megalomania*
Grundbedürfnis: *basic need*
Grundsubstanz: *basic substance*
Grundwert: *basic value*
gurgeln: *gargle*
Gürtelrose: *shingles*
gutartig: *benign*
Gynäkologe: *gynaecologist*

H

Haarausfall: *hair loss*
halluzinieren: *hallucinate*
halluzinogen: *hallucinogenic*
Halluzination: *hallucination*
Hals-Nasen-Ohren-Arzt: *ENT – ear, nose and throat specialist*
Haltung: *posture*
Hämoglobin: *haemoglobin*
Hämorrhoiden: *haemorrhoids*
Harnausscheidung: *diuresis*
Harnröhre: *urethra*
Hasenscharte: *harelip*
Haushaltsplan, Haushaltsmittel: *budget*
Haushaltsunfall: *domestic accident*
Hausmittel: *household remedy*
Hausstauballergie: *house dust allergy*
Haut: *skin*
Hautfarbe: *skin colour*
Hautkrankheit: *skin disease*
Hautausschlag: *skin rash*
Hautblase: *blister*
Hebamme: *midwife*
heilbar: *curable*
heilen: *heal*
verheilt: *healed*
Heilmittel: *remedy*
Heilung: *cure-all*
heiser: *hoarse*
heiß: *hot*
hemmen, stoppen: *arrest*
Herzinfarkt: *heart attack*
Herzstillstand: *cardiac arrest*
Hepatitis: *hepatitis*
Herauslösen, Extrahieren, ziehen: *extraction, extract*

Herpes: *herpes*
hervortretend: *protruding*
Herz: *heart*
Herzschlag: *heart attack*
Herzversagen: *heart failure*
Herz-Lungen-Maschine: *heart-lung-machine*
Herzfrequenz: *heartrate*
Herzklappe: *heart valve*
Herzklappenprothese: *heart valve prosthesis*
Herzschrittmacher: *pace-maker*
Heterosexualität: *hetero-sexuality*
Heuschnupfen: *hay fever*
Hexenschuss: *lumbago*
Hilfe: *help*
hinunterspülen: *wash down*
Hirntod: *brain death*
Histamin: *histamine*
Hitze: *heat*
Hitzschlag: *heat stroke*
HIV-positiv: *HIV positive*
Hodensack: *scrotum*
Höhenangst: *fear of heights*
Homöopathie: *homeopathy*
homöopathisch: *homeopathic*
Homosexualität: *homosexuality*
homosexuell: *homosexual*
hören: *hear*
Hörapparat: *hearing aid*
Hormon: *hormone*
Hornhaut: *cornea*
Hornhaut: *callosity*
Hörrohr: *ear trumpet*
Hörrohr: *stethoscope*
Hüfte: *hip*
Husten: *cough*
Hygiene: *hygiene*
hygienisch: *sanitary*
Hypnose: *hypnosis*
hypnotisieren: *hypnotise*
Hysterie: *hysteria*

I

Idealgewicht: *ideal weight*
im Rausch, betrunken: *ine-briated*

im Reagenzglas: *in vitro*
immun: *immune*
impfen, immunisieren: *immunise*
Impfstoff: *vaccine*
Impfung: *vaccination*
impfen: *vaccinate*
Implantat: *implant*
Impotenz: *impotence*
impotent: *impotent*
Infantilismus: *infantilism*
infiziert: *infected*
Infusion: *infusion*
inhalieren: *inhale*
Injektionsnadel: *cannula*
inkohärent: *incoherent*
inkompatibel, unverträglich: *incompatible*
Inkontinenz: *incontinence*
Inkubationszeit: *incubation period*
Inlay: *inlay*
Innenohr: *inner ear*
instabil: *unstable*
Insulin: *insulin*
Intensivpflege: *intensive care*
internist: *internal specialist*
Intoxikation: *intoxication*
intravenös: *intravenous*
Inzest: *incest*
Iris: *iris*
Ischiassyndrom: *sciatica*

J

japsen, nach Luft schnappen: *gasp*
Jetlag: *jetlag*
Jod: *iodine*
Juckreiz: *itchiness*
jucken: *itch*
Jugend: *adolescence*
Jungfernhäutchen: *hymen*

K

Kabeltransplantat: *cable graft*
Kahlheit: *baldness*
Kahlköpfigkeit: *calvities*
kalkhaltig; verkalkt: *calcareous*
kalorienarm: *low calorie*

kalorienbewusst: *calorie-conscious*
Kalziämie: *calcaemia*
Kalziumausscheidung im Urin: *calciuria*
Kammer: *camera*
Kanal: *canal*
kanalförmig: *canalicular*
Karies: *caries*
Karzinom, bösartige Geschwulst: *carcinoma*
Kauen: *mastication*
kauen: *masticate*
Keim: *germ*
keimfrei: *aseptic*
Keuchhusten: *whooping cough*
Kiefer: *jawbone*
Kieferorthopäde: *orthodontist*
Kinderheilkunde: *paediatrics*
Kinderklinik: *paediatric clinic*
Kinderarzt: *paediatrician*
Kinderkriegen: *have a baby*
Kinderlähmung: *poliomyelitis*
Kindstod: *cot death*
Kissen: *pillow*
Klappe: *valve*
Klappenöffnung: *valve orifice*
Kleinkindalter: *infancy*
Klinge: *blade*
Knie: *knee*
Kniebänder: *knee ligaments*
Kniegelenk: *knee joint*
Kniekehle: *hollow of the knee*
Kniescheibe: *knee cap*
Knöchel: *knuckle*
Knochen: *bone*
Knochenablagerung: *bone deposit*
Knochenbruch: *bone fracture*
Knochendeformität: *bone deformity*
Knochenerweichung: *bone softening*
Knochengewebe: *bone tissue*
Knochenknorpel: *bone cartilage*
Knochenkrebs: *bone cancer*
Knochenmark: *bone marrow*
Knochenmarktransplantation: *bone marrow transplantation*

Knochenschwund: *bone loss*
Knochenwachstum: *bone growth*
Knollennase: *bulbous nose*
Kochsalzlösung: *saline solution*
Kodein: *codeine*
Koffeinmangelmigräne: *caffeine-withdrawal headache*
Koffeinvergiftung: *caffeinism*
Kolibakterien: *coliform bacteria*
Kolik: *colic*
Kolostomie: *colostomy*
Koma: *coma*
komatös, in tiefer Bewusstlosigkeit: *comatose*
Komparative Psychologie: *comparative psychology*
Komplikationen: *complications*
Kompresse : *compress*
Konservenvergiftung: *can poisoning*
Konsiliararzt: *consultant*
Kontaktlinse: *contact lens*
Kontrastmittel: *contrast medium*
Kontusion, Prellung: *contusion*
Kopf: *head*
Kopfhaut: *scalp*
koronare Herzkrankheit: *coronary heart disease*
Körper: *body*
Körperflüssigkeit: *body fluid*
Körperöffnung: *body orifice*
Körperhaltung: *body posture*
Körperempfinden: *body sense*
Körpergewicht: *body weight*
Körperbehinderung: *physical disability*
Kräfteverfall: *cachexia*
kraftlos, schwach: *feeble*
Krampf: *cramp*
Krampfader: *varicose vein*
Krankenbericht: *medical record*
Krankenbett: *sick bed*
Krankengeld: *sick benefit*
Krankengymnastik: *physical therapy*
Krankenhaus: *hospital*
Krankenschwester: *nurse*
Krankentrage: *stretcher*

Krankenwagen: *ambulance*
Krankheit: *illness*
Krankschreibung: *sick leave*
kratzen: *scratch*
Kraut: *herb*
Kräutermedizin, Kräuterheilkunde: *herbal medicine*
Krebs: *cancer*
krebsartig: *cancerous*
Kribbelgefühl: *prickling feeling*
Krise: *crisis*
kritisch: *critical*
Krücke: *crutch*
Kugelgelenk: *ball-and-socket joint*
Kugelprothese: *ball-and-socket prosthesis*
Kunstfehler: *malpractice*
künstlich: *artificial*
künstliche Befruchtung: *artificial insemination*
künstliche Beatmung: *artificial respiration*
Kürrettage, Ausschabung: *curretage*
Kurzatmigkeit: *shortness of breath*
kurzsichtig: *shortsighted*
Kurzzeitgedächtnis: *short-term memory*

L

Labor: *laboratory*
Lackmus: *litmus*
Lähmung: *paralysis*
Laken, Bettlaken: *sheet*
lallen: *babble*
Langlebigkeit: *longevity*
Laparoskopie: *laparoscopy*
Laser: *laser*
Lasertherapie: *laser therapy*
Latex: *latex*
Laus: *louse*
Leben: *life*
Lebenserwartung: *life expectancy*
leblos: *lifeless*
lebenslang: *lifelong*
lebensbedrohlich: *life-threatening*

Lebensmittelvergiftung: *food poisoning*
lebensrettend: *lifesaving*
Leber: *liver*
Leberblindpunktion: *blind liver biopsy*
Lebertran: *cod-liver oil*
Legalisierung: *legalisation*
Leiche: *corpse*
Leichenstarre: *cadaveric rigidity*
Leichnam: *cadaver*
leicht verletzt: *slightly injured*
Leiste: *groin*
Leprakranker: *leper*
Lepra: *leprosy*
Lernstörung: *learning disorder*
Lese-Rechtschreibstörung, Legasthenie, Dyslexie: *dyslexia*
Lethargie: *lethargy*
Leukämie, Blutkrebs: *leukaemia*
Leukozyt: *leucocyte*
Lezithin: *lecithin*
Libido: *libido*
Lichttherapie: *phototherapy*
liegen: *lie*
lindern: *alleviate*
Linolsäure: *linoleic acid*
Linse: *lens*
Lipid: *lipid*
Liposom: *liposome*
Lippe: *lip*
Lippen lesen: *lip-read*
lispeln: *lisp*
Logopädie: *logopaedics*
löslich: *soluble*
Luftröhre: *trachea*
Luftröhrenschnitt: *tracheotomy*
Lumbalpunktion: *lumbar puncture*
Lungenentzündung: *pneumonia*
Lutschtablette: *pastille*
Lymphknoten: *lymph node*
lymphatisches System: *lymphatic system*
Lymphgefäße: *lymphatic vessels*

M
Magenkrebs: *cancer of the stomach*

masturbieren: *masturbate*
medizinische Wissenschaften, Heilkunde: *medical science*
Misshandlung: *maltreatment*
Müdigkeit: *fatigue*
Multiple-Sklerose: *multiple sclerosis*
Mumps: *mumps*
Mundgeruch: *bad breath*
Mund-zu-Mund-Beatmung: *mouth-to-mouth resuscitation*
Muskel: *muscle*
Muskelkrampf: *muscle cramp*
Muttermal: *birth mark*
Muttermilch: *mother's milk*
Myopie: *myopia*

N
Nabel: *navel*
Nabelbruch: *umbilical hernia*
Nabelschnur: *umbilical cord*
Nachlässigkeit: *negligence*
nachtblind: *night-blind*
Nachtdienst: *night duty*
Nachtschwester: *night nurse*
Nacken: *neck*
nackt: *naked*
Nadel: *needle*
Nagel: *nail*
Nagelbett: *nail bed*
nähen, vernähen: *stitch (up)*
Nährstoff: *nutrient*
Naht: *suture*
Narbe: *scar*
Narbengewebe: *scar tissue*
Narkose: *narcosis*
Narkotikum, Rauschgift: *narcotic*
Narzissmus: *narcissism*
nasal: *nasal*
Nasenhöhle: *nasal cavity*
Nasenspiegelung: *nasoscopy*
Nase: *nose*
Nasenbluten: *nosebleed*
Nasenloch: *nostril*
Nasentropfen: *nose drops*
Naturheilkunde: *naturopathy*
natürlich: *natural*
Nebenhoden: *epididymis*
Nebenwirkungen: *side effects*

Nerv: *nerve*
Nervensystem: *nervous system*
Nervenzusammenbruch: *nervous breakdown*
Nesselsucht: *nettle rash*
Netzhaut: *retina*
neugeboren: *newborn*
Neuralgie: *neuralgia*
Neurodermitis: *neurodermatitis*
Neurologie: *neurology*
Neurologe: *neurologist*
Neurose: *neurosis*
neurotisch: *neurotic*
Neurotiker: *neurotic*
Nickelallergie: *nickel allergy*
niedriger Blutdruck: *hypotension*
Niere: *kidney*
Nierenversagen: *kidney failure*
Nierenstein: *kidney stone*
niesen: *sneeze*
Nikotin: *nicotine*
Notfall: *emergency*
Notruf: *emergency call*
Notoperation: *emergency operation*
Notstation: *emergency ward*
nüchtern: *with empty stomach*
Nymphomanie: *nymphomania*
Nymphomanin: *nymphomaniac*

O

Oberarm: *upper arm*
Oberbegriff für die medizinischen Berufe: *medical profession*
Oberschenkel: *femur, femoral*
Ödem: *oedema*
offene Herzchirurgie: *open-heart surgery*
öffentliches Gesundheitswesen: *public health*
ohnmächtig werden: *faint*
Ohr: *ear*
Ohrensausen: *buzzing*
Onanie: *masturbation*
Onkologie: *oncology*
Onkologe: *oncologist*
Operation: *operation*
Operationssaal: *operating theatre*

Organ: *organ*
Orthopädie: *orthopaedics*
Orthopäde: *orthopaedist*
örtlich: *local*
Osteoarthritis, Gelenkentzündung, Osteoporose: *osteoporosis*
Östrogen: *oestrogen*
Ovulation: *ovulation*

P

Palliativ: *palliative*
palpabel: *palpable*
Palpitation: *palpitation*
Panik: *panic*
Pap-Abstrich: *pap smear*
paradontose: *periodontosis*
Paraffinöl: *liquid paraffin*
Paranoia: *paranoia*
Paranoiker: *paranoiac*
Parkinson-Krankheit: *Parkinson's disease*
Patient: *patient*
Penis: *penis*
peptisch: *peptic*
pericardial: *pericardiac*
Pericarditis: *pericarditis*
Periode: *period*
Periodenschmerz: *menorrhalgia*
Peristaltik: *peristalsis*
Pessar: *pessary*
Pflegeheim: *nursing home*
Pickel: *pimple*
Pigment: *pigment*
Pille: *pill*
Pilzerkrankung: *fungal infection*
Plasma: *plasma*
Plazebo: *placebo*
Plazenta: *placenta*
Plombe, Füllung: *filling*
Pollen: *pollen*
Pollenallergie: *pollen allergy*
Polyp: *polyp*
privat, Privat-: *private*
Privatpatient: *private patient*
Probe: *sample*
Probe: *specimen*
Prognose: *prognosis*
Prostata: *prostate*

Prostatismus: *gland prostatism*
Psychiater: *psychiatry*
Psychologie: *psychology*
psychisch: *psychological*
Pubertät: *puberty*
Pufferlösung: *buffer solution*
pulmonal: *pulmonary*
Puls: *pulse*
Pulsfrequenz: *pulse rate*
Pupille: *pupil*

Q
Quarantäne: *quarantine*
Querschnittslähmung: *paraplegia*
Querschnittsgelähmter: *paraplegic*
quetschen: *crush*

R
Rachitis: *rickets*
Radiographie: *radiography*
Radiotherapie, Strahlentherapie: *radiotherapy*
Raucherhusten: *smoker's cough*
Rasterelektronmikroskop: *scanning electron microscope*
Reflex: *reflex*
Reflexhandlung: *reflex action*
regenerieren: *regenerate*
Rehabilitation: *rehabilitation*
Rehabilitationszentrum: *rehabilitation centre*
reif: *mature*
Remission: *remission*
rezeptfrei: *over-the-counter*
Rhesusfaktor: *Rhesus factor*
Rheumatismus: *rheumatism*
Riechnerv: *olfactory nerve*
Rinderwahn: *mad cow disease*
Rippe: *rib*
Risikogeburt: *high risk delivery*
Risswunde, Einriss: *laceration*
Rollenspielen: *roleplaying*
Rollstuhl: *wheelchair*
Röteln: *German measles*
Rückbildung: *atrophy*
Rücken: *back*
Rückenschmerzen: *backache*
Rückfall: *relapse*
Rückfluss: *regurgitation*

Rückgrat, Wirbelsäule: *spine*
Rückstand: *residue*
Ruhe: *rest*

S
Salbe: *ointment*
Salmonella: *salmonella*
Salzmangel: *salt depletion*
Samen: *sperm*
Samenbank: *sperm bank*
Samenerguss: *ejaculation*
Samenleiter : *deferent duct (sperm duct, vas deferens)*
Samenleiterdurchtrennung: *vasectomy*
Sanatorium: *sanatorium*
Säugen, Stillzeit: *lactation*
stillend: *lactating*
Saugflasche: *feeding bottle*
Säuglingsnahrung: *babyfood*
Saugreflex: *sucking reflex*
Säure: *acid*
Säure, Säuregrad: *acidity*
Scanner: *scanner*
Schädel: *skull*
Schädeldecke: *skull cap*
Schädelkapsel: *cranium*
schädlich: *harmful*
Schamhaar: *pubic hair*
Scharlach: *scarlet fever*
Scharlach: *canker rash*
Scharniergelenk: *hinge joint*
Scheide: *vagina*
Scheidenabstrich: *vaginal smear*
Scheidenspiegelung: *vaginoscopy*
Scheidewand: *septum*
Schere: *scissors*
Schicht: *shift*
Schichtarbeit: *shift work*
schielen: *squint*
Schienbein: *shinbone*
Schienbein: *tibia*
Schiene: *splint*
Schilddrüse: *thyroid*
schizophren: *schizophrenic*
schlafen: *sleep*
Schlaf: *sleep*
Schlaftablette: *sleeping pill*

Schlafkrankheit: *sleeping sickness*
schlaff: *flabby*
Schlaflosigkeit: *insomnia*
Schläfrigkeit, Müdigkeit: *drowsiness*
schläfrig: *drowsy*
Schlaganfall: *stroke*
schlank: *slim*
Schlauch: *tube*
schleimabsondernd: *mucous*
Schleimhaut: *mucous membranes*
Schleim: *mucus*
Schluckauf: *hiccough*
Schluckimpfung: *oral vaccination*
Schlund: *pharynx*
Schmerz: *pain*
Schmerzzentrum: *pain centre*
Schmerzmittel: *painkiller*
schmerzlos: *painless*
Schmerzlinderung: *painrelief*
Schmerzgrenze: *pain threshold*
Schmetterlingsbruch: *butterfly fracture*
Schmetterlingswirbel: *butterfly shaped vertebrae*
schnarchen: *snore*
Schneidezahn: *incisor*
Schnittwunde: *cut*
Schock: *shock*
Schönheitschirurgie, plastische Chirurgie: *plastic surgery*
Schönheitsfehler: *blemish*
Schönheitsfleck: *beauty spot*
Schonkost: *bland diet*
Schorf: *scab*
Schrunde, Fissur: *fissure*
Schulmedizin: *traditional medicine*
Schulter: *shoulder*
Schulterblatt: *shoulder blade*
Schultergelenk: *shoulder joint*
Schuppen: *dandruff*
Schussverletzung: *gunshot wound*
Schutz-: *prophylactic*
Schutzimpfung: *prophylactic*
schwach: *weak*
schwanger: *expectant*
Schwangerschaft: *pregnancy*
schwanger: *pregnant*

Schwangerschaftserbrechen: *morning sickness*
Schwangerschaftsstreifen: *stretchmarks*
Schwellung, Anschwellung: *swelling*
schwerwiegend, schwer: *severe*
Schwindelgefühl: *dizziness*
schwitzen: *sweat*
seekrank: *seasick*
Seekrankheit: *seasickness*
Sehne: *tendon*
Sehnerv: *optic nerve*
Sektion, Leichenuntersuchung: *cadaver dissection*
Selbsthilfegruppe: *self-help group*
Selbstmord begehen: *commit suicide*
Selbstmord: *suicide*
selbstmörderisch: *suicidal*
senil: *senile*
sensibel, empfindlich: *sensitive*
Sensibilität, Empfindlichkeit: *sensitivity*
Sexualtrieb, Geschlechtstrieb: *sensitive*
sezieren: *dissect*
siamesische Zwillinge: *Siamese twins*
sich verbreiten, sich vermehren, wuchern: *proliferate*
sich von einer Krankheit erholen: *to convalence*
Sinusitis: *sinusitis*
Skalpell: *scalpel*
Skorbut: *scurvy*
Sonnenstich: *sunstroke*
spastisch: *spastic*
Spastiker/in: *spastic*
Speichel: *saliva*
Speiseröhre: *oesophagus*
Spender: *donor*
Spenderleiche: *cadaver donor*
spenden: *donate*
Spina Bifida: *spina bifida*
Sprechstunde: *consulting hours*
Spritze: *syringe*
stabilisieren: *stabilise*
stammeln: *stammer*

stationärer Patient: *in-patient*
Stationsarzt: *ward physician*
Stauung: *congestion*
steif, ungelenkig: *stiff*
Steißbein: *coccyx*
steril: *sterile*
sterilisieren: *sterilise*
Stillzeit: *nursing period*
Stress: *stress*
Stuhl: *stool*
Stuhlgang: *bowel evacuation*
Symptom: *symptom*
Syndrom: *syndrome*
Syphilis: *syphilis*

T

Tagesdosis: *daily dose*
Taille: *waist*
Taktfrequenz: *audio-frequency*
Talg: *sebum*
Tampon: *tampon*
Tastsinn: *tactile sense*
Tätowierung: *tattooing*
taub: *deaf*
taubstumm: *deaf-mute*
Taucherkrankheit: *caisson
   disease*
Tee: *tea*
Teer: *tar*
teilnahmslos: *listless*
Teilnahmslosigkeit: *listlessness*
Teint: *complexion*
Telepathie: *telepathy*
telepathisch: *telepathic*
Temperatur: *temperature*
Tennisarm: *tennis elbow*
Thrombozyt: *thrombocyte*
Thrombose: *thrombosis*
Tinktur: *tincture*
Tod: *death*
tödlich: *lethal*
tödliche Dosis: *lethal dose*
Tollkirsche: *belladonna*
Tomogramm: *tomogram*
Tomographie: *tomography*
Tonikum: *tonic*
Totenschein: *death certificate*
Totgeburt: *stillbirth*
tot geboren: *stillborn*

Tourniquet: *tourniquet*
Toxämie: *toxemia*
träge: *lethargie*
Trakt: *tract*
Träne: *tear*
Tränensack: *tear sac*
Tränendrüse: *lacrimal gland*
Transfusion: *transfusion*
Transplantation: *transplantation*
Transplantat: *transplant*
transsexuell: *transsexual*
Traubenzucker: *dextrose*
Trauer: *grief*
Trauerfall: *bereavement*
Trauma: *trauma*
traumatisch: *traumatic*
Tremor, Zittern: *tremor*
Trieb: *instinct*
Tripper: *gonorrhoea*
trocken: *dry*
Tropenkrankheit: *tropical
   disease*
Tropenmedizin: *Tropical
   medicine*
Tropf: *drip or drip-feed*
Trümmerbruch: *complicated
   fracture*
Tuberkulose: *tuberculosis*
Tumor: *tumour*
Typhus: *typhoid fever*

U

übel: *sick, bad*
Übelkeit: *nausea*
überaktiv: *hyperaktiv*
Überaktivität: *hyperactivy*
Überanstrengung: *overstrain*
Überbein: *ganglion*
Überbiss: *overbite*
überdehnen: *distend*
überdehnen: *overstrain*
Überdehnung: *distension*
Überdosierung: *overdosage*
Überdosis: *overdose*
Überdruckbeatmung: *pressure
   breathing*
Überdruckkammer: *hyperbaric
   chamber*
überempfindlich: *hypersensitiv*

Überempfindlichkeit: *hypersensitivity*
Überentwicklung: *overdevelopment*
Überernährung: *superalimentation*
Übererregbarkeit: *erethism*
Überfunktion: *hyperfunction*
Überfunktion der Schilddrüse: *overactive thyroid gland*
Übergangspunkt: *junctional point*
übergeben: *erbrechen*
Übergewicht: *excess weight*
übergreifen: *expand, spread*
Überkompensation: *overcompensation*
Überkorrektur: *overcorrection*
überkreuzen: *cross*
überleben: *survive*
überreif: *overripe*
Übersäuerung: *acidosis*
überschwellig: *supraliminal*
Überstand: *overhang*
Überwachung, Kontrolle: *observation*
übler Mundgeruch: *cacostomia*
Ullrich Turner Syndrom: *Turner's syndrom*
Ulotomie: *incision into the gums*
Ultraschallbild: *sonogram*
Ultraschalluntersuchung: *ultrasound examination*
Ultrazentrifuge: *ultracentrifuge*
Umbildung: *transmutation*
Umhüllung: *velament*
Umlauf: *panaris*
umschneiden: *circumcise*
umstülpen: *invert, turn outside*
Umwelteinfluss: *environmental*
unauffällig: *not contributory*
unbedenklich, sicher: *safe*
unbehaglich, unbequem: *uncomfortable*
unbeweglich: *immobile*
unbewusst: *unvoluntary*
unblutig: *bloodless*

undifferenziert: *undifferentiated*
unehelich: *illegitimate*
unfähig: *incompetent*
Unfall: *accident*
Unfallstation: *first-aid station*
unfruchtbar: *infertile*
ungeboren: *unborn*
Unfruchtbarkeit: *sterility*
ungefährlich: *harmless*
ungehemmt: *uninhibited*
ungesund: *unhealthy*
ungiftig: *non-toxic*
unheilbar: *incurable*
unhygienisch: *unhygienic*
unkompliziert: *simple*
unmündig: *under age*
unreif: *immature*
unsauber: *unclean*
unschädlich: *innocuous*
unsicher: *doubtful*
Untätigkeit: *inertia*
untauglich, ungeeignet: *unfit*
Untauglichkeit: *unsuitability*
unter dem Normalgewicht: *underweight*
Unterarm: *forearm*
Unterbauchregion: *hypogastric region*
Unterbewusstsein: *subconscious*
unterdrücken: *suppress*
unterentwickelt: *underdeveloped*
unterernährt: *undernourished*
untersuchen: *examine*
Untersuchung: *examination*
Untersuchungsbefunde: *clinical examination data*
Untersuchungsmaterial: *specimen*
unverdaulich: *indigestible*
Unverdaulichkeit: *indigestibility*
unverdünnt: *undiluted*
unversorgt: *unattended*
unwillkürlich, vegetativ: *involuntary*
unwohl: *unwell*
Unwohlsein: *malaise*

unzurechnungsfähig: *of unsound mind*
Urin: *urine*
Urinkultur: *urine culrure*
Urintrübung: *cloudiness of the urine*
Urologe: *urologist*
Urologie: *urology*
Uterus: *womb, metra*

V

Vaginalzäpfchen: *vaginal suppository*
Vagus: *vagus*
Vakuummassage: *vacuum massage*
Vakzine: *lymph*
Vaterschaft: *fatherhood*
Vaterschaftstest: *paternity test*
Vegetarier: *vegetarian*
vegetarisch: *vegetarian*
Vehikel: *excipient*
Vene: *vein*
Venenblut: *venous blood*
Venenerweiterung: *venectasia*
Venenpunktion: *venepuncture*
Venenschmerz: *phlebalgia*
Venenstripping: *vein stripping*
Venentransplantation: *vein grafling*
venös: *venous*
Ventilator: *ventilator*
Ventrikel: *ventricle*
verabreichen: *administer*
verängstigt: *scared*
Veranlagung: *disposition*
Veranlagung: *predisposition*
Verband: *bandage*
Verband: *dressing*
Verbandmull: *gauze*
Verbandtasche: *medical wallet*
Verbesserung: *improvement*
verbinden: *bandage, dress*
verbluten: *bleed to death*
verbreiten: *spread*
Verbrennung, Brandwunde: *burn*
Verbrennungsgrad: *burn depth*
Verbrennungsofen: *incinerator*
Verbrennungsschock: *burn shock*
verbrühen: *scald*

Verdacht: *suspicion*
verdauen: *digest*
verdaulich: *digestible*
Verdauungsstörung: *indigestion*
Verdauungtrakt: *digestion*
Verdichtung: *consolidation*
Verdopplung: *doubling*
verdünnen: *dilute*
verdunsten: *evaporate*
vereitern: *suppurate*
verengen: *stenose*
Verengung: *narrowing*
vererbbar: *hereditary*
vererbt: *inherited*
Vererbung: *hereditary factor*
Verfall: *decay*
verfälschend: *falsifying*
verfault: *putrid*
verfettet: *adipose*
verformt, verkrümmt: *deformed*
Verformung, Missbildung, Verkrümmung: *deformity*
verfügbar: *available*
Verhalten: *behaviour*
verhaltensgestört: *disturbed*
Verhaltensmuster: *behaviour pattern*
Verhaltensstörung: *behaviour disturbance*
Verhaltensweise: *behaviour patterns*
Verharren: *perseveration*
verhärten: *harden*
verheilen: *heal*
verhungern: *starve*
Verhütung: *contraception*
Verhütungsmittel: *contraceptive*
verkabeln: *connect up*
verkalken: *calcify*
verkapseln: *capsule*
Verkeilung: *impaction*
verkleben: *adhere*
Verklebung: *adhesion*
verklumpen: *clump*
verknöchern: *ossify*
verknüpfen: *knot, tie*
verkohlen: *carbonize*
Verkohlung: *carbonization*

Verkrümmung: *arcuation*
verkrüppelt: *crippled*
verkrusten: *incrust*
verkümmern: *atrophy*
verlagern: *shift*
verlängern: *lengthen*
Verlangsamung: *slowing down*
Verlauf: *course*
verlegen: *obstruct*
verletzen: *injure*
verletzt: *hurt, traumatized*
Verletzungsgrad: *severity of injury*
Verletzungspotential: *demarcation*
Vermehrung: *reproduction*
Verminderung: *lessening*
veröden: *sclerose*
verordnen: *prescribe*
verrenken: *dislocate*
Verrenkung: *dislocation, luxation*
verrückt: *crazy, mad*
Versagen: *failure*
verschärfen: *aggravate*
verschlechtern: *deteriorate*
verschlechtern: *make worse*
verschleiern: *cloud*
verschleimt: *congested with phlegm*
verschleppen: *spread*
verschließen: *close*
verschlimmern: *make worse*
verschlingen: *devour*
verschlossen: *closed*
Verschluss: *occlusion*
Verschlusskapazität: *closing capacity*
verschmelzen: *fuse*
Verschmutzung: *soiling*
verschreibungspflichtig: *available on prescription only*
Verspannung: *tension*
Verstand: *mind*
Verstärkung: *strengthening*
verstauchen: *sprain*
Verstauchung: *sprain*
Verstopfung: *constipation*

verstreuen: *scatter*
versuchsweise: *probationary*
Verteilung: *distribution*
Vertiefung: *impression, fossa*
Verträglichkeit: *compatibility*
Verwachsung: *union, closure*
Verweiblichung: *effeminization*
Verweildauer: *retention time*
verwesen: *decompose*
verwirrt: *confused*
verwunden: *wound*
verwurmt: *verminous*
verzagt: *despondent*
Verzögerung: *latent period*
verzweigen: *branch*
Vibrationsempfinden: *appreciation of vibrations*
vielgestaltig: *multiform*
Vierfachimpfstoff: *tatravaccine*
Virusisolierung: *virus isolation*
virustötend: *virucidal*
Visite: *visit*
vital: *vigorous*
Vitamin: *vitamin(e)*
Vokalsprache: *vocal speech*
Völlegefühl: *sense of fullness*
völlig: *profound*
Vollwerternährung: *high-quality-nutrition*
voraussagen: *prognose*
Vorbehandlung: *pretreatment*
Vorbelastung: *preload*
Vorbote: *prodrome*
Vorfall: *prolapse*
Vorgeburt: *veil*
vorgeburtlich: *prenatal*
Vorgerinnung: *preclotting*
Vorhaut: *prepuce*
Vorherrschen: *prevalence*
Vorhof...: *atrial*
Vorhof: *atrium*
vorklinisch: *preclinical*
Vormilch: *colostrum*
Vorschrift: *prescription, recipe*

Vorsorgemedizin: *preventive*
Vorsteherdrüse: *prostata*
vorstülpen: *protrude*
vortäuschen: *simulate*
Vorwehen: *false pains*
vorzeitig: *premature*

W

wachsen: *grow*
Wachstumsstörung: *growth disturbance*
Wachzustand: *wakefulness*
wackelig: *wobbly*
Wade: *calf*
Wadenbein: *calf bone*
Wadenbein: *fibula*
Wadenmuskel: *calf muscle*
Wahn, Wahnvorstellung: *delusion*
wahrnehmbar: *perceptible*
Wahrscheinlichkeit: *probability*
Wand: *paries*
wandernd: *migratory*
Wange: *cheek*
Wangenspalte: *genal cleft*
wanken: *stagger*
Wärmebehandlung: *therapeutic use of heat*
Warteliste: *waiting list*
Warteraum: *waiting room*
Warze: *wart*
Warzenvorhof, Inflammation rund um einen Pickel: *areola*
Waschzwang: *ablutomania*
Wasser: *water*
Wassereinlagerung: *water*
Wasserheilkunde: *hydriatics*
Wasserkopf: *hydrocephalus*
Wasserkur: *water cure*
Wasserstoff: *hydrogen*
Wasserzyste: *hydrozyst*
Watte: *cotton wool*
Wattebausch: *cotton swab*
Wechseljahre: *menopause*
Weckmittel: *analeptic*
Wehe: *contraction*
Wehen, Geburt: *labour*
Wehen: *contractions*
Wehen: *labour pains*

Wehenanregung: *induction of labour*
Weisheitszahn: *wisdom tooth*
Weiterbehandlung: *further treatment*
Weitsichtigkeit: *farsightedness*
Wespenstich: *wasp sting*
widerstandsfähig, resistent: *resistant*
wiederbeleben: *resuscitate*
Wiederbelebung: *resuscitation*
Wiederbelebungsversuch: *attempt at resuscitation*
Wiedereinpflanzung: *reimplantation*
Windel: *nappy*
Windeldermatitis: *nappy rash*
Windpocken: *chickenpox*
Wirbelsäule: *vertebral column*
wirksam: *effective*
Wirkung: *effect*
Wismut: *bismuth*
Wissenschaft: *science*
Wochenbettpsychose: *postnatal depression*
Wohlbefinden: *well-being*
Wortfindungsstörung: *amnesic aphasia*
Worttaubheit: *word deafness*
wund: *sore*
Wundermittel: *miracle drug*
wundgelegene Stelle: *bedsore*
würgen: *retch*
Wurmfortsatz: *caecal appendage*
Wutanfall: *tantrum*

X

X-Beine: *knock-knees*
Xanthopsie: *yellow vision*
Xerose: *dryness of a tissue*

Z

Zahn: *tooth*
Zahnarzt: *dentist*
Zahnarzthelferin: *dental assistant*
Zahnbrücke: *bridge*
Zähne: *teeth*
Zahnen: *teething*
Zahnentzündung: *dental infection*

Zahnextraktion: *tooth extraction*
Zahnfleischentzündung: *gingivitis*
Zahnlücke: *gap*
Zahnmedizin, Odontologie, Zahnheilkunde: *odontology*
Zahnprothese, Gebiss: *denture*
Zahnschmelz: *enamel*
Zahnschmerzen: *toothache*
Zahnspange: *brace*
Zahnstein entfernen: *scale*
Zahnstein: *plaque*
Zahrarztstuhl: *dentist's chair*
Zange: *forceps*
Zangengeburt: *forceps delivery*
Zartheit: *tenderness*
Zecke: *tick*
Zeckenenzephalitis: *tick-borne*
Zehe: *toe*
Zehnagel: *toenail*
Zeichensprache: *sign language*
Zeigefinger: *index finger*
Zellentwicklung: *cytopoiesis*

Zerfall: *decay*
zittern: *quiver*
Zucken: *twitching*
zucken: *twitch*
zugelassen: *approved*
zulassen: *approve*
zurechnungsfähig: *sane*
zurückfließen: *regurgitate*
zurückgeblieben: *retarded*
zurückkehren: *regress*
zusammenbrechen: *break down*
Zusammenbruch: *breakdown*
Zusatzstoff: *additive*
zustimmen: *consent*
Zwang: *compulsion*
Zwangseinweisung: *compulsory hospitalisation*
Zweibeiner: *biped*
Zweistärkenbrille: *bifocal glasses*
Zwerchfell: *diaphragm*
Zwillinge: *twins*
Zwillingsforschung: *gemellology*
Zyste: *cyst*
Zystenausschneidung: *cystectomy*